The Home Care Companion's

QUICK TIPS FOR CAREGIVERS

The Home Care Companion's

QUICK TIPS FOR CAREGIVERS

Marion Karpinski, R.N.

Medifecta Healthcare Training
Medford, Oregon

Printed in Canada

Cover Design: Robert Frost Design

Illustrations:
Don Thomas, pages 4, 21, 24, 25, 26, 37, 45, 46, 48, 49, 50, 51, 55, 57, 59, 61, 62, 66, 80, 86, 115, 145, 155, 157, 158, 161, 165, 180, 183.
Ernie Hinchcliffe, pages 11, 33, 38, 56, 75, 77, 83, 91, 98, 119, 123, 129, 141, 172, 185.
Laura Burkhalter, window illustration at chapter beginnings, and pages 69 and 110.

Library of Congress Cataloging-in-Publication Data
Karpinski, Marion 1948-
        The Home Care Companion's Quick Tips for Caregivers
    p.   cm. 5
ISBN 0-9653873-9-9
1.Caregivers--United States 2. Aged--Care--United States

✸ DEDICATION

Dedicated to all the families and caregivers who over the years continue to inspire me.

✸ ACKNOWLEDGEMENTS

My sincere thanks and appreciation to all those who so willingly helped me with research, editing, proofreading, and professional support in the development of this book. To Gaea Yudron, Jim Lamberson, Robin Emmens, M.S., Ann Close, R.N., Cynthia Alvarado, R.N., Mary Hall, R.N., Rosy Thomas, O.T., Bev Bowman, R.N., E.T., Arline Borella, R.N., Kurt Wilkening, O.D., deputy fire marshall Roy Brown, audiologist William Strock, and a special thanks to my husband Mike for his loving support.

DISCLAIMER: This book is published for educational purposes only, and is not intended to take the place of medical diagnosis and treatment.

TABLE OF CONTENTS

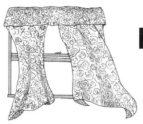 # Preface

The love we give away is the only one we keep.

∼ ELBERT HUBBARD ∼

I have worked with many patients and families in my 30 year career as a registered nurse. During my lifetime, many changes have occurred in the way health care is delivered. In the past, nurses were the primary caregivers. We provided most of the nursing care in the hospital, and in many ways we discouraged families from participating in providing care. We knew that most families didn't have the experience or medical background to provide the sophisticated level of care needed. During a time of seemingly unlimited resources, there was no reason to burden families with work we could do ourselves.

The situation is quite different now. Several years ago, as part of an attempt to lower health care costs, there was a shift from hospital care to home care that had significant impact on patients and their families. Today, patients are being discharged from the hospital much more quickly, some still requiring nursing care. Visits made by home care nurses are helpful, but even those visits are limited in time and frequency.

Family caregivers are taking over many functions and duties previously provided by hospitals and nurses. Skills we nurses take for granted are major challenges for family caregivers. Unprepared family members find themselves anxious and frustrated because they do not have the knowledge or skills needed to provide care.

I wanted to help families acquire those skills. I wrote and directed a video specifically designed for family caregivers. It was very well received by hospices, hospitals, and home health agencies across the country. People who used the video found it provided the skills they needed and reduced personal anxiety, giving them the confidence to provide the most loving kind of home care. The positive response we received, along with requests for other video programs, inspired us to continue. Now there are eight videos in *The Home Care Companion Video Collection*, with several more in the planning stages.

This book, *The Home Care Companion's Quick Tips For Caregivers*, is designed as a friendly tool for family caregivers to use during their daily caregiving routine. *Quick Tips* provides a wide variety of information and resources. Having the knowledge to perform basic

caregiving procedures safely builds confidence and provides an opportunity for both caregiver and family to
experience the deeper rewards of caregiving.

Marion Karpinski, R.N.
Director, Healing Arts Communications

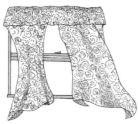

Introduction

*The capacity to care is the thing which gives life
its deepest meaning and significance.*

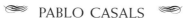 PABLO CASALS

Being a Caregiver Today

Few people eagerly look forward to the day when they can finally become caregivers. Most of us dread taking up the demands of caregiving, anticipating that it will mean profound sacrifices. Yet, when the time arrives, we usually assume the caregiving role with a great deal of grace. As family members, we recognize that we may be the ones best equipped to provide emotional and spiritual support for our relatives. Giving care can also be seen as a way of serving and repaying loved ones for the care and love they have given us.

Caregiving today is different from what it was in the past. We are responsible to our jobs, our children require our support and guidance, and at the same time we are caring for our elderly parents. Not only are more of us growing older, but the diseases that afflict us are medically managed for longer periods of time. Alzheimer's disease, Parkinson's disease, multiple strokes, and dementia are examples of progressive diseases that can require years of caregiving.

Being accountable for a family member's health and well being is a big responsibility. Family caregivers often lack emotional detachment because of their relationship to the other person. They may lose a sense of themselves as individuals, become overly involved, and become emotionally depressed or physically ill. This doesn't have to happen.

Giving until there is nothing left to give is not successful caregiving. You need not sacrifice your own health or emotional balance to ensure that your loved one survives. Caregiving involves establishing effective emotional boundaries, setting reasonable limits on your work, and developing a certain amount of loving detachment from your family member's ongoing health condition. Caregiving today includes learning how to take care of yourself, accepting the fact that you can't do it alone, and acquiring the knowledge and skills needed to provide care.

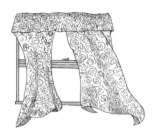

Chapter 1
Prepare Yourself and Your Home

You will serve as a medical advocate for the person in your care, and that means you will be a very important part of your family member's health care team. Don't be intimidated by doctors or nurses. Be assertive. Let your voice be heard!

- Establish an open communication with the doctor. Make sure you understand the medical condition clearly. If you don't understand something the doctor says, speak up immediately and ask for clarification.

- Don't settle for a relationship with a physician that is not satisfactory for you or your loved one. It is your right to have a physician who is sensitive to your needs and takes the time to answer your questions.

❧ Prepare a written list of questions about the details of care you will be expected to provide, and take notes whenever you are with the doctor or nurse. You may find it useful to be able to refer to your notes later.

❧ Accept the fact that you can't do everything yourself. This is a time when teamwork and cooperation are vital. Don't be shy about asking for help. In many ways, your own health and well being as a caregiver will depend upon the support of others.

❧ Before your family member leaves the hospital, make a list of caregiving tasks such as grocery shopping, meals, laundry, housecleaning, medical appointments, and errands. When someone offers to help, he or she may not know how to be of help. Don't leave it up to the other person to figure out how to contribute. Give him or her a way to participate. Suggest one or two items on the list with the times when that help is needed.

❧ Volunteer help may be available through your church or community agencies.

Before Hospital Discharge

❧ Develop a working relationship with the case manager or discharge planner. Case managers are a wealth of information. The case manager can connect you to services available in your community and answer questions about insurance coverage, financial concerns, and acquiring in-home help.

🍂 Set up an information center near the main phone in the house that contains medical and emergency information.

Include:

- Medicare and insurance policy numbers.
- A list of existing medical problems.
- A list of all medications currently being taken.
- The primary doctor's name and phone number.
- The address and phone number of your home. Other caregivers may not remember this information in an emergency.
- A note pad to write down information or instructions.

🍂 Show other caregivers the information center and the type of information available there.

🍂 Learn CPR and the Heimlich Maneuver. You can take a course in these emergency procedures at low cost through the American Red Cross or your local hospital.

🍂 Plan some time during each day that is just for you. Caregiving can be overwhelming. You can prevent caregiver burnout by making a plan before your family member is discharged from the hospital.

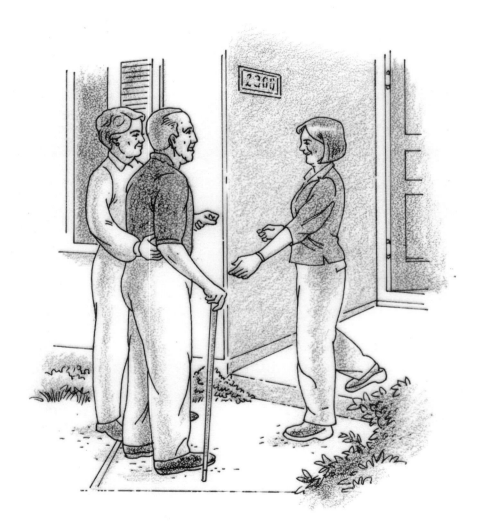

Coming Home from the Hospital

🌿 You should receive a list of current medications at the time of discharge. Be sure you understand the purpose of each drug, how to give each medication, and possible side effects. Do not continue an old medication routine without first checking with the nurse or doctor.

🌿 Prioritize your caregiving tasks. The person will be tired when he or she gets home from the hospital. You may feel tired yourself. Make an outline showing which tasks will need immediate attention and which tasks can wait.

🌿 You may also receive a list of all the home care supplies you will need. Make sure you know where they can be purchased.

Home Medical Equipment

🌿 Using specialized home medical equipment can make caregiving tasks simpler and safer. If you haven't recently been in a home medical supply store, you may be surprised. In the past, home medical supply stores were extensions of the hospital. Today they are more like retail stores geared toward helping family caregivers. Browse through the store to see if there are any products that can help you. New equipment is being designed every day to help empower families and make caregiving easier. Talk with the store's knowledgeable staff, who can answer your questions. Ask for help in making decisions about any equipment with which you are not familiar.

☙ Other outlets for purchase of medical equipment include pharmacies, medical supply catalogs, department stores, and hospitals.

☙ Prices vary, and prescriptions are necessary for insurance coverage. HMOs contract with particular vendors.

☙ Home medical equipment can also be borrowed or rented from The Red Cross, Salvation Army, Visiting Nurses' Association, home care agencies, charity organizations, churches, and senior centers.

☙ Before you buy medical equipment, get recommendations from your health care professionals or from the hospital discharge planner.

☙ Seek out dealers with a good reputation for service.

☙ Be sure to follow instructions for safe installation. Most home medical equipment suppliers can deliver, install, and teach you how to use equipment properly.

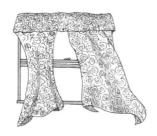

Chapter 2
Home Care Services

We make a living by what we get,
but we make a life by what we give.

❦ SIR WINSTON CHURCHILL ❦

The three major types of home care services available are skilled care, custodial or supportive care, and hospice care. Medicare, private health insurance, and some long term care insurance plans may pay for these services. State programs may pay for medical services for low income and disabled persons. Check with your state senior or disabled services or your state health plan. Check the insurance plan of the person for whom you are caring to see what home care benefits are available.

Skilled Care

Skilled care must be ordered by the doctor. Skilled care requires that a professional nurse or therapist perform some skilled function, such as changing dressings, wound care, medications, bowel and bladder training, and physical or speech therapy. Skilled care is paid for by Medicare only if the patient is homebound. Homebound means that it is physically taxing or unsafe for the person to leave home. As long as skilled care is required, Medicare will also pay for a home health aide to perform personal care such as bathing or showering. The personal care aide must be discontinued when skilled care is no longer needed.

Custodial or Supportive Care

- Custodial or supportive care is defined as personal care tasks such as bathing, showering, being assisted to the bathroom, light housekeeping, and meals.

- Medicare does not pay for this type of service. Custodial or supportive care is often an out-of-pocket expense. Some private health insurance and long term care insurance plans have in-home care benefits that pay for custodial or supportive care. Some state health plans pay for this service.

Hospice Care

- Hospice care is for people with a limited life expectancy. Hospice nurses provide symptom management, emotional support, and grief counseling, working with the family as well as the patient.

✿ Hospice services must be ordered by the doctor.

✿ Hospice care is covered by Medicare, some state health plans, and private insurance plans.

Respite Care

The word respite means relief, vacation, breather, pause, or time off. Respite care is necessary for all caregivers, and is provided by professional and informal caregivers.

✿ Respite care can be in-home or outside the home. An informal caregiver such as a church volunteer, friend, or relative may come to the home to relieve the primary caregiver. A professional caregiver may provide relief at an adult day care or respite center. The person is taken to the center for several hours, providing free time for the caregiver.

✿ Find out more about respite opportunities in your area by contacting:

• Community services in the phone directory

• Your local Area Agency on Aging

• Respite and adult day care centers

• State senior and disabled services

• Your church

How to Hire a Caregiver through a Home Care Agency

✿ Home care agencies provide skilled services, hospice care, and custodial or supportive care. Some agencies provide only skilled services, or only custodial or supportive services.

🍃 Using a home care agency may cost more per hour than hiring a private duty caregiver, but the agency can save you time and frustration.

🍃 The home care agency recruits, evaluates, hires, disciplines, bonds, and pays the aide, substitutes another aide because of illness or vacation, files necessary government forms, and pays employee taxes.

Before you choose an agency:

🍃 Interview several agencies.

🍃 Find out how long the agency has been in business.

🍃 Is the agency Medicare-certified?

🍃 Ask if employees are bonded. Do they run a criminal check and drug testing on potential employees?

🍃 What are the qualifications and training of the aides?

🍃 What are the complete costs?

🍃 Find out how you will be billed. Who bills the insurance?

🍃 You can find a home care agency by checking the Yellow Pages under nursing services, senior services, social services and your local Area Agency on Aging.

How to Hire a Private Duty Caregiver

🌿 Hiring someone to assist with caregiving at home requires careful planning and follow-through.

🌿 As the employer, you are responsible for finding, evaluating, hiring, disciplining, finding a substitute aide because of illness or absence, payroll and employee taxes, and mandatory government tax forms.

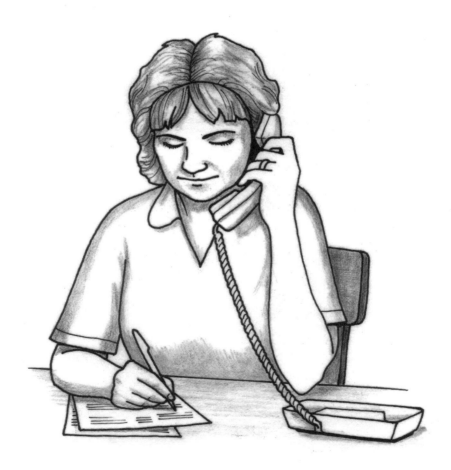

❧ For tax information, ask the Internal Revenue Service for the Household Employer's Tax Guide or call your local social security office. For state tax information, contact your state employment department.

❧ Write a job description that includes the daily needs and preferences of the person for whom you are caring. Include any problems such as incontinence, confusion, and behavior problems. List personal care tasks such as bathing and exercising, and household tasks such as vacuuming, shopping, meal preparation, and laundry.

❧ Write down the daily or weekly frequency of each task. Determine the number of hours you will need someone to work each week and the hourly wage.

❧ A thorough job description will help applicants understand what is required of them and can help you hire the right person.

Sources for finding a private duty caregiver include:

• Friends, family members, co-workers, and members of your support group. Word of mouth is often the best place to start.

• A hospital case manager or discharge planner

• Hospital senior services

• Local or state Area Agency on Aging office/ Eldercare Locator

- Your church or synagogue, Catholic Charities, Jewish Family Services
- The Yellow Pages under nurses, nursing services, senior services, and social services
- State or county social services department
- The American Red Cross
- Schools of nursing

🌾 Screen candidates by telephone. Ask each applicant the same questions. These are some of the questions to ask:

- Are you licensed or certified?
- What is your caregiving experience?
- Have you taken classes or training to prepare for this work?
- Are you able and willing to perform all the job duties?
- When are you available to start work?
- Is the hourly rate I am willing to pay acceptable?
- How long have you lived in this area?
- Why did you leave your last job?
- Can you provide at least three references from families you have cared for in the past?
- Have you recently taken a drug test or had a criminal background check?
- Are you a smoker or non-smoker?

❦ From your initial phone screening, select the best qualified people and schedule a personal interview with each of them. The person being cared for should be present at the personal interview, if possible.

❦ During the interview, evaluate the applicant's personality, work history, personal appearance, health, and communication skills.

❦ Present a complete list of the tasks you expect the person to perform, and discuss job duties.

❦ If the job duties involve driving, ask to see the applicant's driver's license and registration. You can ask applicants to supply a DMV record showing their driving record for the last 2-3 years.

❦ After the interview, always check at least three references. Remember that you will be trusting this individual with your loved one. Even if you feel good about the person, you must check references to be absolutely sure that this person is as he or she appears.

When you contact the references given by the applicant, be sure to ask them:

❦ How long have you known the applicant?

❦ Did the applicant work for you? If so, would you hire him or her again?

❦ Is he or she dependable and trustworthy?

🌿 How does the applicant handle conflicts and emergencies?

🌿 Does the applicant work well independently?

🌿 Do you have anything else you would like to say about the applicant that I haven't asked you?

🌿 Run a criminal background check. If the person has been a state resident for some time, the state police (and in some cases Senior Services) will provide this information. Otherwise, it must come from the FBI, and can take months.

🌿 When you have selected an applicant, create a written agreement that specifies and records all the agreed upon issues. Be sure you and the hired caregiver both date and sign the agreement. A signed agreement will help to resolve any misunderstandings that may arise in the future. The agreement should specify job duties, hours and days, wage, payday, auto reimbursement, whether or not meals will be provided, smoking, dress code, TV, radio, visitors, telephone use, and termination notice required by you and the hired caregiver.

Geriatric Care Management

As the caregiver of an elderly relative, you may not feel comfortable with all the decision making that is required. Your job and children may need your attention. If your elderly relative lives a long distance from your community, caregiving can be more difficult because of the separation. In addition, you may not know what services are available in his or her community.

Geriatric care managers can be a great help in these situations. The care manager is a registered nurse or social worker. He or she assists clients and their families with long term care needs. The services of a geriatric care manager are often covered by long term care insurance or private pay. Some of the services available are physical, mental, psychological, environmental, and financial assessments. The care manager can arrange in-home and volunteer services, assist with alternative living placements, identify cost-effective community services, assist with transportation needs, schedule and accompany the elderly person to doctor appointments, help with difficult decisions, such as whether the elderly person is still a safe driver, monitor physical and mental needs, and keep families informed with regular reports on the elder's status.

To locate a geriatric care manager, contact your local Area Agency on Aging office or senior and disability services. The National Association of Professional Geriatric Care Managers has a website where you can learn more about geriatric care managers. The site, (www.caremanager.org), also lists care managers in each state. The organization can be reached by phone at (520)881-8008.

RECOMMENDED READING

When Aging Parents Can't Live Alone, Ellen F. Rubenson, 2000, Lowell House, Los Angeles.

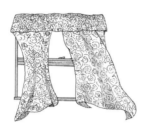

Chapter 3
The Importance of Communication

Laughter is the shortest distance between two people.

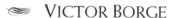

VICTOR BORGE

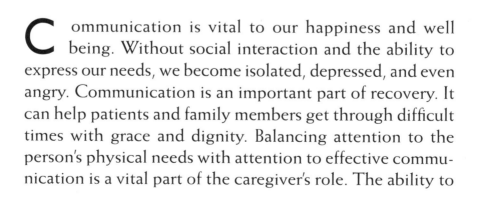

C ommunication is vital to our happiness and well being. Without social interaction and the ability to express our needs, we become isolated, depressed, and even angry. Communication is an important part of recovery. It can help patients and family members get through difficult times with grace and dignity. Balancing attention to the person's physical needs with attention to effective communication is a vital part of the caregiver's role. The ability to communicate differs widely according to a person's physical and mental capabilities. These basic guidelines and techniques can help to develop more positive, effective communication.

General Tips for Good Communication

- ❧ Continue to treat the person as a mature adult. Speaking to a person in a condescending or belittling way, as if he or she were a child, brings on tension and resentment.

- ❧ Observe the other person's body language and facial expressions. Listen to his or her tone of voice for the feelings it expresses.

- ❧ Communicate nonverbally through eye contact, posture, and gestures, indicating that you are interested in what is being said. Be aware of your own body language. Body language that conveys frustration, impatience, or anger gives a stronger message than your words.

- ❧ Use touch as a way of offering encouragement and support. Each person has different comfort levels when it comes to being touched. Be sensitive to individual preferences.

- ❧ Try to listen to everything, not just what you want or expect to hear.

- ❧ Move the person you are caring for to a window or an area of activity such as the living room or kitchen, where stimulation and communication are more likely to occur. Include the person in discussions about family matters and in conversations.

🕊 Initiate conversation. Look out the window and comment on the weather or something going on outside. Read a newspaper headline out loud and make a comment. Ask a question about a favorite personal possession or an activity the person is interested in.

🕊 Speak in a natural tone of voice. Don't assume that speaking louder will help the person to understand better, unless he or she is hearing impaired.

How to Communicate Effectively with Someone Who Has Hearing Loss

🕊 Never start a conversation from another room. Go to the person and get his or her attention before you begin to speak.

🕊 Minimize distractions such as radio or TV sounds or the sound of other conversations.

🕊 Face the person and maintain eye contact, unless eye contact is culturally inappropriate.

🕊 Speak from a position 3-6 feet away, with your face at eye level.

🕊 Avoid sitting with your back to a window or a light source. Your face will be poorly lit, and the glare from the light behind you will make it difficult for the listener to see your face and mouth.

🕊 Speech reading refers to the way we receive cues about what is being said through lip movements, facial expression, body postures, and gestures. We all speech read to some degree. People with hearing loss rely more heavily on speech reading. Chewing gum, smoking, or covering your mouth while talking hides important visual cues and should be avoided.

- If you speak quickly, slow down. Otherwise, speak at your normal pace. Speak every word clearly without exaggerating. Exaggerating your lip movements makes facial cues hard to understand.

- Never speak directly into the person's ear. This can distort your message.

- Speaking slightly louder than usual can be helpful, but avoid shouting. Shouting can distort your message and make you appear to be angry.

- If the person does not understand what is being said, rephrase the sentence using different words that may be more easily understood.

- When you are communicating something important, ask the person to repeat what you've just said, or write down the information to make sure he or she understands you.

- Make sure the person's hearing aid is in place before you begin care. Loss of communication, even for short periods of time, can bring feelings of helplessness and frustration.

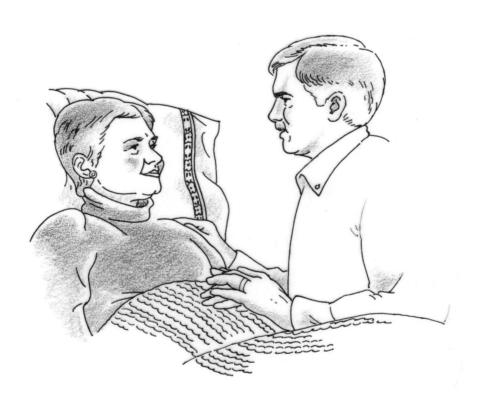

The Role of Understanding

The loss of control over many familiar areas of life leaves many older people feeling confused, angry, or unneeded. Understanding your loved one's physical, emotional, and mental experience will help you to maintain tolerance and empathy.

🌿 Honoring your loved one's perspective and innate need for dignity will open the way for more effective, loving communication.

🌿 Understanding your own emotions is also important. Most caregivers feel some resistance, fear, anger, frustration, and guilt doing the work of giving care. Finding creative ways to work with tensions and difficult emotions can provide opportunities for personal growth.

🌿 Finally, understand your family's needs. Maintain an open dialogue with family members. Allow time for family activities and excursions. Family cooperation and participation makes giving care a positive shared experience.

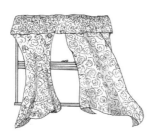

Chapter 4
Taking Care of the Caregiver

Light is the task where many share the toil.

 HOMER

Stress

Stress is part of life and caregiving can be particularly stressful. We can't eliminate stress in our lives, but we can learn to recognize and manage it. One of the best ways to manage stress is to become aware of the earliest warning signs. Our bodies tell us when we are having stress. We need to listen to our bodies. Only you know your earliest warning signs of stress. Learn them and pay attention to them. If you ignore the early warning signs and wait until

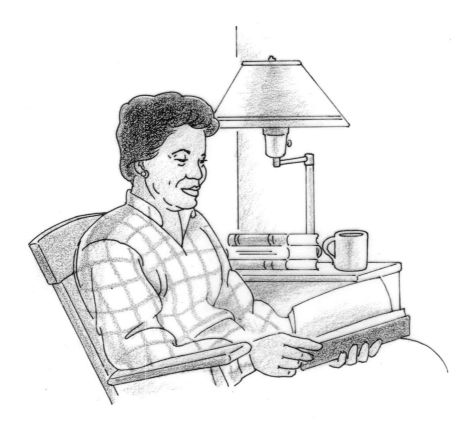

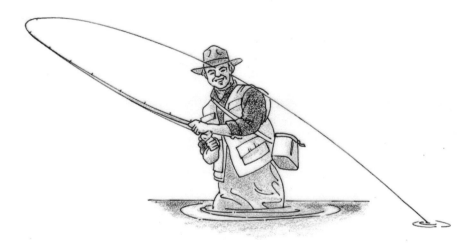

stress becomes severe, it is much harder to regain your se-renity.

Tips to Help Reduce Stress

Here are some tips for self-care that can help reduce stress, enhance your well being, and increase your energy.

☙ Acknowledge your feelings. Caregivers often feel conflicting emotions. Try sitting quietly, practicing meditation, prayer, or meditative movements such as yoga or tai chi. Quiet moments like these can help you listen to your inner voice and get in touch with your feelings.

- Find ways to share what you feel with friends, clergy, family members, or counselors.

- Release stress by stretching. Step outside and breathe deeply. Look at the sky. Listen to music that makes you happy.

- Find something to laugh about. Laughter reduces stress by stimulating breathing and increasing muscular activity and heart rate. Laughter is like an internal body massage.

- Make time for regular exercise—at least 20 minutes, two or three times a week.

- Eat a healthy diet. Eat regular meals. Don't skip breakfast. Drink plenty of water!

- Get 6-8 hours of uninterrupted sleep every night. Rejuvenate during the day by taking short naps.

- Get a massage. Swim. Dance. Work in the garden. Go for a walk or go to a movie.

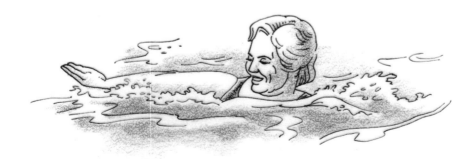

🍂 Schedule regular dental and medical appointments for yourself.

🍂 Guard against infections by maintaining good personal hygiene. Bathe daily, wash hands thoroughly and often, and apply moisturizing creams to your skin.

🍂 Don't try to be "superman/woman." Set realistic goals.

🍂 Use professional and informal respite care and other community resources.

🍂 Delegate jobs to friends and family members who are willing to help.

Releasing Difficult Feelings

As a caregiver, you may have to deal with unpleasant or frustrating situations that bring up difficult feelings in you such as anger, sadness, guilt, or helplessness. You can use these methods for releasing difficult feelings before they reach crisis level.

🍂 Accept the fact that there are some things you can't change. Change only the things you can.

🍂 If you are sad or angry, allow yourself to cry. Your emotions are natural. Let yourself feel them without guilt.

🍂 Live one day at a time.

🍂 Use positive self talk. Slogans such as "Easy does it," "First things first," and "How important is it?" can help turn a negative day into a positive one.

🍂 Start a gratitude list. There is always something for

which we can be grateful. Start with the alphabet and for each letter think of something for which you are thankful.

🌿 Join or start a caregiver support group where you can share your feelings with others and learn from others' shared experiences.

🌿 Learn as much as you can about your loved one's disease. It will help you to have realistic goals for that person. Remember, you didn't cause the disease and you can't cure it or control it.

🌿 Avoid destructive behaviors such as using drugs or alcohol, overeating, or outbursts of anger.

🌿 Prioritize your tasks and do only those that really need to be done.

🌿 Release your anger by going for a walk, writing in your journal, or yelling into or punching a pillow, rather than holding your feelings in or taking them out on others.

Warning Signs of Increasing Stress

🌿 Ongoing irritation or edginess.

🌿 Loss of interest in social activities.

🌿 Intense fear and anxiety about money or the future.

🌿 Fatigue or recurring physical problems such as backaches, headaches, or lingering cold or flu symptoms.

🌿 Difficulty concentrating.

🌿 Lethargy or depression.

❦ Feeling overwhelmed.

❦ Increasing use of alcohol, overeating, or use of drugs in order to relax.

❦ Feeling trapped or hopeless.

❦ Thoughts of suicide, thoughts of violence, or actual acts of physical violence against the person for whom you are caring.

Don't ignore these red flags, for your own sake and the sake of the person for whom you are caring. Services are available in the community that can help. Here are some places to look for a support group or counselor:

- Area Agency on Aging
- Hospital senior services
- The community services section in the phone directory
- The counselor's section in the phone directory. Ask for a referral to a counselor who has experience with caregivers
- Religious service agencies, clergy, or parish nurses
- Community health or mental health clinics
- Newspaper: Check the "events calendar" for support group meetings

RECOMMENDED READING

The Caregiver Helpbook: Powerful Tools for Caregiving, Vicki L. Schmall, Ph.D., Marilyn Cleland, R.N., Marilynn Sturdevant, R.N., M.S.W., L.C.S.W., 2000, Legacy Caregiver Services, Portland, OR. (503)413-6578

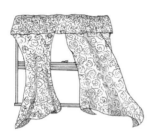

Chapter 5
Infection Control

Germs are harmful microorganisms that can cause disease and infection. The goal of infection control is to limit the spread of germs and to prevent them from causing infection and disease to you and the person for whom you are caring.

How Germs are Spread

Direct Contact

Any time you touch someone who is sick, you are in direct contact. Bathing, handling any body fluid such as sputum, urine, or stool, or changing dressings are examples of direct contact. Colds are often spread by direct contact. When someone sneezes into his hand and later touches another person's hand, the germ is transferred. When that person touches her nose, eyes, or mouth, the cold germ enters the body.

Indirect Contact

Indirect contact is touching objects such as dishes, bed linens, clothing, or equipment that have been in direct contact with someone who is ill.

Airborne Contact and Droplet Transmission

Airborne contact occurs when you breathe in germs carried by dust or droplets that are suspended in the air after someone infected sneezes, coughs, or talks.

Vehicle Spread

Vehicle spread occurs when germs are introduced into your body through contaminated drugs, food, water, or blood products. Diarrhea can be the result of ingesting food or water contaminated with germs.

Vector Spread

Vector spread is the spread of germs from animals or insects. Fleas and rats, for instance, were carriers of the bubonic plague. Today, ticks carry Lyme's disease.

Correct Handwashing

🌿 Handwashing is the single most effective way to reduce the spread of germs.

🌿 It is important that you wash your hands correctly before and after giving care, to protect yourself and the person for whom you are caring.

🌿 Wash your hands before and after touching medical equipment, food, and pets. To wash your hands correctly:

1. Turn the water on and adjust it to a comfortable temperature. Allow the water to run. Angle the hands downward.

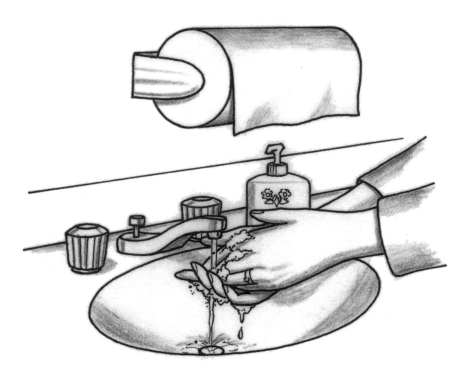

2. Avoid using bar soap. Use a mild, antiseptic soap dispensed from a pump bottle.

3. Wet your hands and apply soap, working up a good lather.

4. Friction helps to mechanically remove germs from the hands. Use a rotating and rubbing motion.

5. Rub every part of the hand: in between the fingers, thumbs, palms, and above the wrists. Wash for at least 10-15 seconds.

6. Clean all the areas of the hands, especially around the fingertips, where we do most of our touching.

7. Wash under rings. Never remove jewelry before washing and replace it after washing. You are putting germ-contaminated jewelry right back on your clean hands. Avoid wearing ornate jewelry with grooves where germs can lodge.

8. Use a nail brush for cleaning under the nails.

9. Rinse thoroughly, holding your hands downward under the running water. Start at the wrists and rinse to the fingertips.

10. Use clean paper towels to dry your hands.

11. Use another paper towel to turn off the faucet. Avoid touching the faucet handles or sink with your clean hands.

12. Apply lotion after washing to keep your skin from becoming dry and chapped.

Protective Barriers

You can prevent germs from entering your body by wearing protective barriers, including gloves, aprons or gowns, masks, and protective eye wear.

Gloves

Gloves that are used to protect us from germs are often made of latex and are intended to be used one time only. Disposable gloves are often referred to as exam gloves. Disposable gloves used as a barrier against germs come in a box similar to a tissue box.

Wear gloves:

- When taking a rectal temperature.
- When cleaning someone after a bowel movement.
- When removing soiled dressings or linens.
- When touching equipment that may have body fluid on it.
- When handling all body fluids.
- A good rule of thumb is: if it's wet, wear gloves.
- Always use new gloves for each procedure.
- Keep in mind that gloves are not totally safe. Fluids can leak in over the cuff, or a glove may have a hole in it.
- Always wash your hands after you remove gloves.

Putting On and Removing Gloves

- Remove all jewelry from your hands.
- Keep your fingernails short.
- Wash your hands thoroughly.
- Inspect the gloves for tears or perforations.
- Pull the gloves on before providing care.
- To remove gloves, first use the right hand to remove the left glove. Put your right fingers under the left wrist cuff and pull the glove downward until it is off. The glove will be turned inside out. (See illustration)
- While holding the left glove in your right hand, insert the thumb or two fingers of your left hand into the cuff of the right glove. Do not touch the outside of the glove with your bare hand.
- Pull the right glove down. It will be inside out and the left glove will be within it.
- Dispose of both gloves in an appropriate container.
- Wash your hands.

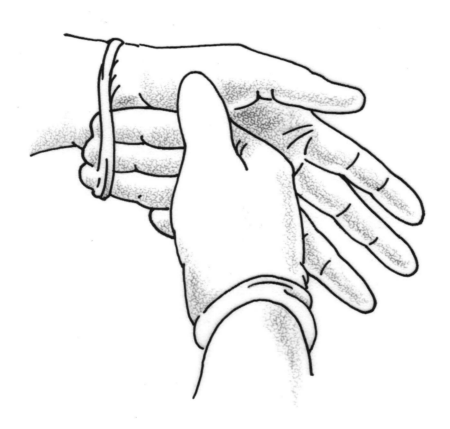

Gowns or Aprons

- Protect your clothing and skin by wearing an apron or smock. Disposable aprons are available through home medical supply stores.

- If your clothes become wet with someone's body fluid, remove them quickly, then wash and change into clean, dry clothes.

Masks

Wearing a mask will protect you from breathing airborne germs in through your nose and mouth. Various kinds of masks are available. Some have elastic that wraps around the ears, some go around the head, and some offer additional eye protection.

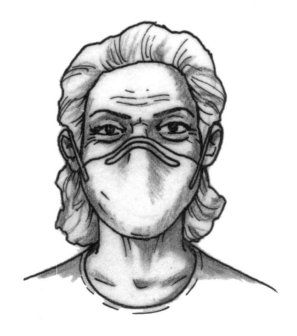

- ❧ The mask should cover your nose and mouth completely.

- ❧ Use a mask when you are working closely with someone who is coughing frequently.

- ❧ Use a mask during suctioning, use of a Water-Pik, or whenever there is a chance of any splashing of body fluid.

- ❧ Change the mask if it becomes moist or wet.

- ❧ Remove the mask when you leave the room. Try to touch only the string tie or elastic. Pull the elastic band from the back of your head to the top. Then lift both elastic bands at the side of your head over your head and remove the mask.

- ❧ Dispose of the mask in an appropriate container.

- ❧ Wash your hands.

Eye Protection

- ❧ Wear eye protection when there is a chance that you could be sprayed or splashed with body fluids.

- ❧ Prescription glasses offer eye protection.

- ❧ If you don't wear glasses, purchase an inexpensive pair of protective glasses.

- ❧ Ask the home care or doctor's office nurse for a source of protective eye wear.

Cleaning the Home

- ❧ Cleaning the home creates an environment conducive to healing.

❧ The living area should be kept clean, orderly, and well ventilated.

❧ Keep the supply table and night stands free of dust. Wipe up spills immediately.

❧ To kill germs, use a disinfectant such as Lysol or Pine-Sol. You can make your own disinfectant solution by using a mixture of one part chlorine bleach to ten parts water. Rubbing alcohol can be used to disinfect small items such as thermometers.

❧ When you are housecleaning, clean the bathroom last.

❧ Movable medical equipment should be cleaned in the bathroom. Then clean the bathroom with a disinfectant. Never reuse a bathroom cleaning cloth or brush to clean another area of the house.

❧ Protect your hands by wearing rubber dishwashing gloves when cleaning. The gloves may be washed and worn again, but should be thrown away if they are peeling, cracked, discolored, or have punctures or tears.

❧ Wash mop heads and dust cloths once a week. Dry them separately in the clothes dryer at the "hot" setting. Dry them before storing in the closet.

Soiled Laundry

❧ Bed linens should be washed at least once a week.

❧ Remove linens from the bed by folding them into quarters to avoid shaking dust and germs into the air. Folding the top blanket into quarters will make it easier to replace without shaking.

❧ Soiled or wet bed linens should be changed and laundered immediately.

❧ Wear gloves and an apron to protect yourself when removing soiled or wet bed linens or clothing.

❧ If you need to carry the soiled laundry through the house, put the laundry in a plastic or cloth bag first.

❧ Wash the soiled or wet linens separately from other family laundry. Dry linens separately and thoroughly on the "hot" setting.

❧ Most laundry detergents are adequate, but for heavily soiled laundry, add a cup of bleach or Lysol to the load.

❧ Use hot water whenever possible. Dry the laundry on the hottest setting, or hang the washed laundry in the sun. The sun is a natural disinfectant.

❧ If you need to hand wash the laundry, use two tablespoons of bleach per gallon of water. Wear rubber gloves. Rinse thoroughly.

Disposal of Body Waste

❧ Body fluids such as urine, feces, and blood may be flushed down the toilet.

❧ Disposable items that contain infectious body fluids such as bed pads or dressings should be wrapped in newspaper first to absorb excess moisture and then placed into a leakproof plastic bag. Tie or twist-tie the bag tightly and dispose of it in the trash.

Storage of Medical Supplies

❧ Store medical supplies in a clean, dry, draft-free area.

❧ Do not store medical supplies on the floor; use a supply table.

❧ Keep medical supplies away from household traffic and protected from dirt, dust, heat, moisture, insects, pets, and children.

❧ A spare bedroom is a good place to store medical supplies. Avoid storing supplies in the bathroom or kitchen.

❧ Have adequate lighting in the storage area.

❧ Check the expiration dates on all medical supplies routinely, and dispose of any medical supplies that are expired.

❧ When new supplies are brought in, bring the existing supplies forward and use them first.

❧ Never use medical supplies that are soiled or damaged.

❧ Previously opened bottles containing sterile solutions should be stored with the caps securely in place. Store them in a cool, dry place away from direct sunlight.

❧ Use a clean bed sheet or plastic sheet to cover stored supplies.

Signs and Symptoms of an Infection

An infection may still develop even when we follow strict infection control guidelines. If you recognize any of the following signs or symptoms of an infection, report them immediately to your doctor or home care nurse:

- Temperature greater than 100 degrees for longer than 48 hours
- Fever, chills, sweating
- Sore throat
- Cough
- A change in the color or amount of sputum
- Burning or painful urination
- Diarrhea
- Nausea
- Vomiting
- Pain or tenderness
- Changes in the skin: redness, rash, hot to the touch, or swelling
- Pus or drainage with an unpleasant odor from a wound or body opening
- Unusual fatigue

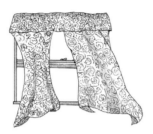

Chapter 6
Daily Home Care Activities

If you find it in your heart to care for someone else,
you will have succeeded.

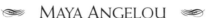 MAYA ANGELOU

Principles of Body Mechanics

Caregiving involves body movements such as lifting, reaching, and bending. You can reduce the risk of injury to your back when you apply the principles of body mechanics: a set of rules that help maintain correct body posture during any movement. Proper posture maintains the natural curves of the spine, helping to conserve energy and prevent muscle strain.

In the standing position, proper posture includes:

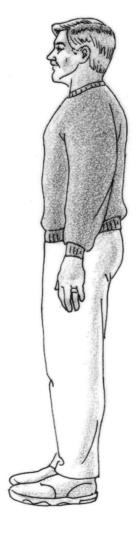

Head erect

Shoulders back and relaxed

Chest up

Arms at sides

Abdomen flat

Buttocks slightly tucked in

Knees unlocked

Feet flat on the floor
and parallel about
12 inches apart

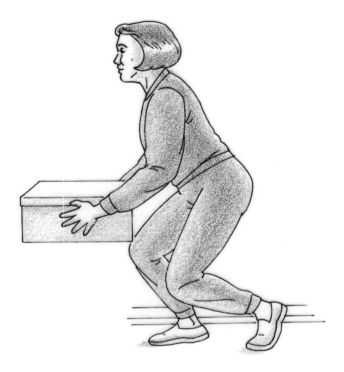

How to Protect Your Back

Lifting

- Think about your body's posture and position before you begin to lift.

- Lift first in your mind, and then with your body.

- Whenever you can, slide, roll, or push instead of lifting. Avoid straining the back muscles by pulling.

- Get as close as possible to the object or person without leaning forward.

- Position your body first. Stand with your feet apart 8 to 12 inches, one foot slightly forward, to make a solid, broad base of support.

- Get down on one knee or squat if necessary so that you are on the same level as the object.

- Keep your back straight. Never bend from the waist.

- Bend your knees when lifting.

- Tighten your stomach muscles and lift, using the strong muscles of your thighs rather than your back.

- Always lift in a smooth motion to prevent injury.

- To change direction, never twist your body at the waist. Instead, take small steps and turn your entire body as a unit in the direction you want to face.

- Set the object down slowly, bending at the knees and keeping your back straight.

Back Safety Tips

- Wear comfortable, non-skid shoes and a back belt to help protect the back when lifting.

- Know your limits and observe them. Be aware of the maximum amount of weight you can lift or move safely.

- When you must stand for long periods of time, put one foot on a foot stool and change position every 20 minutes. This will ease some of the strain on the lower back.

- Avoid reaching for or lifting anything above the head. Try to get on the same level as the object, or use a reacher.

How to Care for Someone on Bedrest

Bedrest Positions

Proper positioning in bed promotes rest and comfort and improves circulation, breathing, and overall body function. There are four basic bedrest positions.

I. Lying on the Back

- Keep the head in line with the body.
- Support the head with a pillow placed under the neck. The pillow should extend from the lower neck to the head. Do not allow the head to fall back.

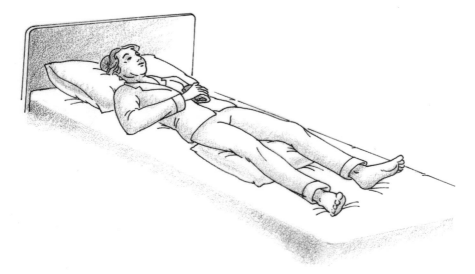

- Keep the knees bent by placing a pillow under them. This will relieve stress on the lower back.
- A rolled washcloth or small towel placed in the hand helps keep the hand from contracting.

❧ A foot board may be required for someone on long term bedrest. The foot board keeps the feet in proper position and prevents "foot drop," a condition that results from the foot remaining in a forward position for extended periods of time.

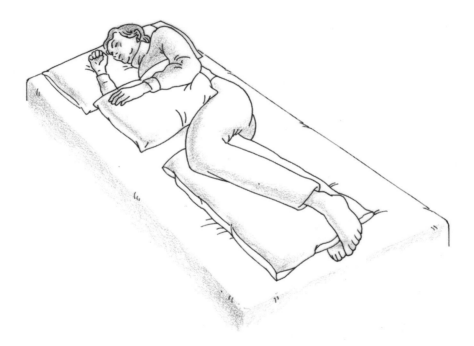

2. Lying on the Side
This position helps relieve pressure on the back.

❧ Support the top leg with a large pillow placed between the legs. Support the entire leg, including the ankle.

❧ The arm under the body should be in front of the chest and bent upward at approximately a 90 degree angle.

❦ Watch the arm under the body for impaired circulation. Reposition the person if he or she complains of numbness, pain, or tingling, if the arm is cool or discolored, or if the fingernails are blue.

❦ Support the upper arm, forearm, and hand with a pillow. The arm should be kept in a bent position, close to the body.

❦ Support the head with a small pillow. Keep the head in line with the spine.

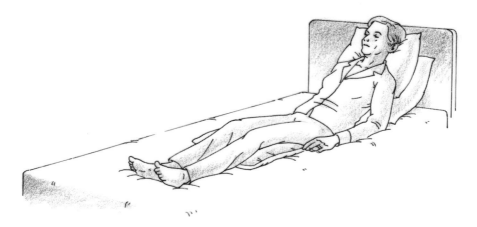

3. Sitting and Modified Sitting

The sitting position does put pressure on the base of the spine and the heels, but can be modified to relieve pressure on those areas.

❦ Bed posture is important. Make sure that the head is in line with the spine and the back is straight.

❦ If you are using a hospital bed, the hips should be at the downward bend of the mattress.

💧 Support the shoulders and head with pillows. The pillows should be placed under the shoulders first. Then position additional pillows under the head.

💧 If you are using a conventional bed, place a small pillow under the knees.

💧 For a modified sitting position, the head of the bed is raised no more than 30 degrees, to reduce pressure to the lower back. A thin pad or pillow is placed under the legs from the mid-calf to the ankle. The heels are elevated slightly to eliminate pressure.

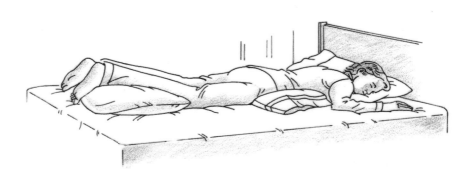

4. Prone (Lying on the Abdomen) and Modified Prone

The prone position can relieve pressure to the back and hip bones. Do not use this position if the person you are caring for has cardiac disorder, respiratory distress, recent abdominal surgery, or if the person complains of discomfort. Most people find the prone position comfortable for only 15-20 minutes.

- Let the feet hang over the edge of the bed in the proper flexed position, and support the ankle joint by placing a folded towel beneath the ankle. You can also position the person with the feet remaining on the bed. In this position you need to place a pillow from the knees to the ankles so that the feet are in a flexed position. Both foot positions help to prevent pressure on the toes and ankles.

- Place a small pillow or folded towel under the abdomen if it increases comfort.

- Turn the head to the side and rest it on a flat pillow, folded blanket, or towel.

- The arms should be at the sides or bent at the elbows toward the head of the bed.

- For modified prone position, bring one knee up toward the chest, placing the opposite arm behind the body. A flat pillow or towel can be placed under the knee, ankle, shoulder or abdomen if this provides more comfort.

How to Move and Position Someone in Bed

Make it a habit to pause and think about the principles of body mechanics before you begin to move or position someone. Plan your move according to what you have learned you can and cannot do.

Tell the person what you plan to do and ask for cooperation and assistance. Let the person do as much of the move as he or she is capable of.

How to Move Someone to the Edge of the Bed

Moving the person to the edge of the bed brings him or her closer to your center of gravity. This will make it easier to move or turn the person into different positions.

- Begin with the bed in a flat position and raised to a height that is level with your elbows. If the bed is not adjustable, you need to lower your body to the level of the bed by bending your knees and keeping your back straight.

- If you are working alone, move the person in sections, starting with the upper body.

- Stand with your feet 8-12 inches apart, one foot in front of the other, as close to the bed as possible, with your knees bent to allow you to shift your weight.

- Slide your arms under the person's shoulder so that your hand reaches to the far shoulder. Slide your other arm underneath the middle of the back until your hand reaches to the far edge of the back. Tense your abdominal and buttocks muscles. Keep your elbows as close to your body as possible.

- Count 1-2-3, and on the count of three, bring the shoulders toward you, sliding your arms along the sheet as you shift your weight from your forward foot to your back foot in a smooth motion. The person's upper body will be on your side of the bed.

- Move the middle body in a similar way. Stand with your feet 8-12 inches apart, one foot in front of the other, close to the bed, knees bent, and slide one arm just below the waist at the hips and the other arm just below the buttocks.

ᴗ Count 1-2-3, and on the count of three, bring the middle body toward you, sliding your arms along the sheet as you shift your weight from your forward foot to your back foot in a smooth motion.

ᴗ Repeat the same procedure for the lower legs, sliding your arms underneath the thighs and the lower legs, bringing the legs and feet in line with the rest of the person's body.

ᴗ If you have someone available to assist you, one person can slide the upper body at the same time that the other person slides the lower body toward the edge of the bed.

How to Move Someone toward the Head of the Bed

ᴗ Tell the person what you are going to do.

ᴗ Begin with the bed in a flat position. Raise the bed to a height that is level with your elbows. If you cannot raise the bed, lower your body to the level of the bed, bending your knees and keeping your back straight.

ᴗ Begin with the person lying flat on her back and remove the pillow or pillows. Place a pillow against the headboard to protect the head when moving up.

ᴗ Ask the person to bend her knees and brace her feet and hands firmly on the bed to help push.

ᴗ Stand with your feet about 12 inches apart, with the

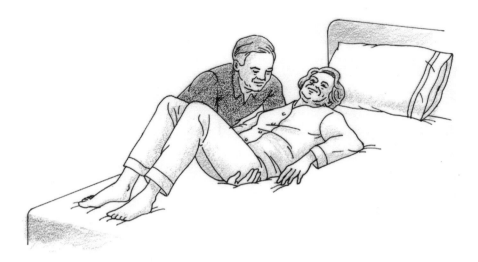

foot that is closest to the head of the bed pointing in that direction.

🌿 Bend your knees and keep your back straight.

🌿 Slide one arm under the shoulders and the other arm underneath the buttocks.

🌿 Count 1-2-3, and on the count of three, have the person push with her feet and hands while you help by sliding her toward the head of the bed with your arms, shifting your weight from your back leg to your front leg in a smooth motion.

🌿 Keep in mind that you can use several small upward moves rather than a single large one to reach the head of the bed.

🌿 Replace the pillow under the head. Check to be sure that her head is in line with the spine.

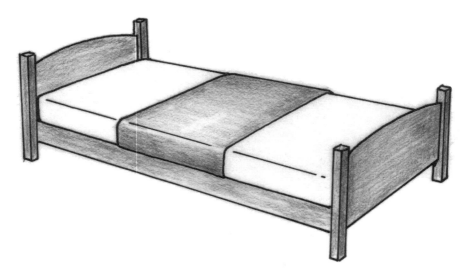

How to Use a Draw Sheet

A draw sheet is an additional sheet folded lengthwise and placed in the middle third of the bed under the person's torso and buttocks. Using a draw sheet, one or two people can more easily slide a person toward the edge or head of the bed.

How to Move Someone toward the Edge of the Bed Using a Draw Sheet

- ❧ The bed should be flat.
- ❧ Loosen the draw sheet on both sides of the mattress. Stand close to the side of the bed, with your feet 8-12 inches apart.
- ❧ Place one foot in front of the other and bend your knees.
- ❧ Roll the draw sheet against the person's side.
- ❧ Grasp the roll firmly, with one hand at the person's

shoulder and one hand at the hip. If the person is heavy, you can move him or her in sections. First the shoulders and chest area, and then the hip area.

🕊 Begin to pull the person toward you, using your legs, not your back, as you shift your weight from your front foot to your back foot in a smooth motion.

How to Move Someone toward the Head of the Bed Using a Draw Sheet

🕊 The bed should be flat. Remove the pillow from under the head. Place the pillow at the headboard to protect the head while moving.

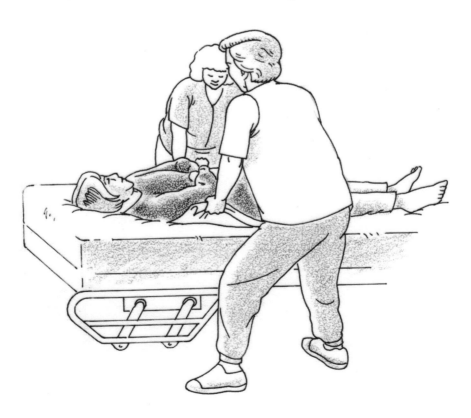

 You will need someone to assist you. Start by stand- ing on opposite sides of the bed.

 Both you and your assistant should stand with feet 8-12 inches apart and your bodies turned slightly to- ward the head of the bed. The foot closest to the head of the bed should point in that direction.

 Together, untuck the draw sheet from both sides of the mattress and roll the draw sheet close to each side of the person's body.

 Bend your knees and keep your back straight. Grasp the rolled sheet.

 Count 1-2-3, and on the count of three, together slide the draw sheet with the person on it smoothly toward the head of the bed, as you shift your weight from your back foot to your front foot.

 After the move is complete, adjust the person's posi- tion if necessary. Replace the pillows under the head. Be sure to smooth the draw sheet until it is free of wrinkles. Tighten it, and tuck it under the sides of the mattress.

How to Raise the Head and Shoulders

 The person should be lying flat, close to the edge of the bed, with his knees bent.

 Stand next to the person, facing the head of the bed, feet 8 to 12 inches apart, one foot in front of the other.

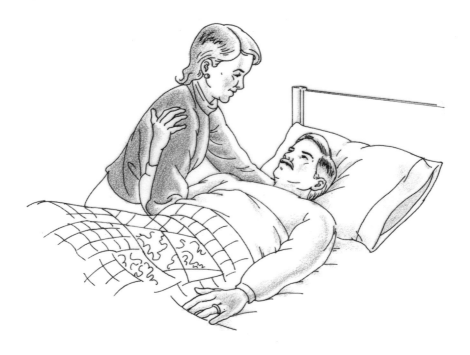

❦ Tell the person what you plan to do. If you need to replace a pillow, have the new pillow ready and within reach.

❦ Place your arm under the person's arm closest to you and brace your hand against the back of his shoulder.

❦ Ask him to put his arm under your arm on the same side and wrap it around your back, bracing his hand against the back of your shoulder.

❦ Slide your other arm under the person's neck and shoulders.

❦ When you're ready, count 1-2-3, and on the count

of 3, raise the head and shoulders from the bed as you shift your weight from your forward foot to your back foot.

☙ Support him at the shoulders and use your other arm to remove or readjust the pillow.

☙ To return the person to the lying position, continue to support him in the locked arm position, supporting the neck and shoulders as you gently lower him down.

How to Help Someone Sit Up at the Edge of the Bed

☙ Tell the person what you are going to do. He should be lying on his side close to the edge of the bed, facing you. If he can, ask him to place his hand flat on the bed in front of his chest and have him use that hand and arm to help push himself up.

☙ Stand at the edge of the bed with feet 12 to 18 inches apart and lower your center of gravity by bending your knees.

☙ Place your hand and arm under the person's knees and slide your other arm under and around the person's back. Assist him into a sitting position by bringing his knees over the side of the bed while lifting his upper body into a sitting position. Be sure to use your legs to lift, not your back.

☙ Remain in front of the person until he is stabilized.

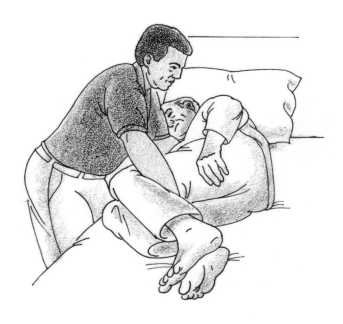

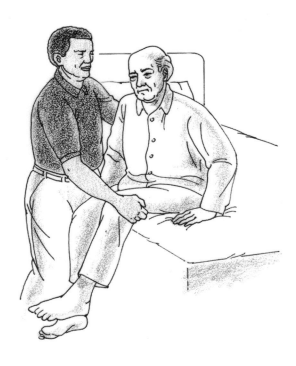

How to Turn Someone on Her Side, Facing You

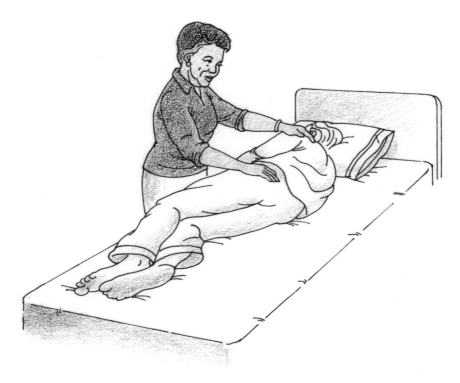

🌿 Begin with the person lying on her back close to the center of the bed, so that after she is rolled toward you, there will be sufficient room for her to lie on her side.

🌿 Stand as close to the bed as possible, feet 8-12 inches apart, with one foot in front of the other and your knees slightly bent.

🌿 Cross the person's leg that is farthest from you over the closer leg.

🌿 Cross her arms over her chest.

- Place your right hand on her farthest shoulder and your other hand on her farthest hip.

- Brace yourself against the side of the bed and gently roll her toward you as you shift your weight from your front foot to your back foot.

- Check the arm under the body. The arm should be in front of the chest, not underneath the body. The elbow should be bent upward at a 90 degree angle toward the head of the bed.

- Place a pillow in front of the chest to support the upper arm.

- Adjust the legs by bending the upper leg toward the chest. Support the entire upper leg, including the ankle, by placing one or more pillows between the legs.

- The back should be straight, and the head in line with the spine.

How to Turn Someone on His Side, Facing Away from You

- If the bed has side rails, raise the rail on the side the person will be facing after the move. If there are no bed rails, place a pillow on that side to prevent the person from rolling off of the bed accidentally.

- Begin with the person on his or her back at the edge of the bed closest to you.

- Stand as close to the bed as possible, with your feet 8-12 inches apart, one foot in front of the other and your knees slightly bent.

🕭 Cross the person's arms over the chest.

🕭 Cross the person's closer leg over the farther leg.

🕭 Place your hand under his near shoulder and the other underneath his buttocks.

🕭 Bend your knees to lower your center of gravity and gently push the person away from you, rolling him onto his side.

🕭 You may need to realign the person's position on the center of the bed. You can do this by sliding your arms under the hips. Shift your weight as you draw the hips toward you, sliding your arms along the sheet. Stop at the center of the bed.

🕭 Adjust the shoulders in the same manner. Place a pillow lengthwise along the back, and tuck it under snugly to keep the person from rolling back. Place a small flat pillow under the head.

🕭 Position the body in the side bedrest position.

How to Move Someone into the Prone Position

🕭 Start with the person lying on his back. Remove the pillow from under the head.

🕭 Move him to the edge of the bed. (refer to page 53)

🕭 Next, turn him on his side, so that he faces the middle of the bed. (refer to page 63)

🕭 Stand at the side of the bed, facing him.

🕭 Straighten the arm that is closest to the mattress, and, with his palm up, tuck the arm under his lower thigh.

🕭 The upper arm should be bent at approximately a 90

degree angle and positioned up towards the center and head of the bed, palm down.

- Bend his upper hip and knee toward you. This will make turning easier.

- Place one hand on the top shoulder and the other on the top hip. As you bend your knees, shift your weight to the back foot and slowly roll the person toward you onto his abdomen.

- Check the head immediately to be sure that he is not face down on the bed or pillow. Move the lower arm from underneath the body and place it at his side, or place the arm toward the head of the bed with the elbow bent.

- Let the feet hang over the edge of the bed in the proper flexed position, and support the ankle joint by placing a folded towel beneath the ankle. You can also position the person with his feet remaining on the bed. In this position you need to place a pillow underneath the legs from the knees to the ankles so that the feet are in a flexed position. Both of these foot positions help to prevent pressure on the toes and ankles. (refer to page 51)

- Place a small pillow or folded towel under the abdomen if it increases comfort.

- Turn the head to the side and rest it on a flat pillow, folded blanket, or towel.

- The arms should either be at the sides or bent at the elbows, hands toward the head of the bed.

Pressure Ulcers (Bedsores)

A pressure ulcer is a breakdown of tissue caused by unrelieved pressure to the skin. Pressure ulcers, also known as bedsores, will occur if a person confined to a bed or wheelchair is not repositioned regularly.

The areas of the body that receive the greatest amount of pressure to the skin are called pressure points. These include the coccyx (tailbone), elbows, knees, heels, head,

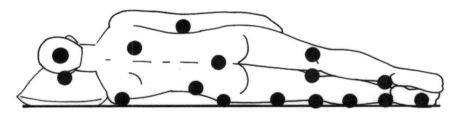

Pressure Points

and buttocks. The skin begins to break down when blood flow is restricted at these pressure points or at any other part of the body.

Pressure ulcers may also develop from friction or shear when moving and repositioning a person. Friction occurs when the skin is rubbed against bed linens. Shear occurs when the pressure of movement pulls the skin in the opposite direction from the movement. One example of shear is when someone slides down in bed. Pressure ulcers may also be caused by inadequate bathing, the person's inability to feel parts of their body, careless handling of the person, or moisture from urine, perspiration, or draining wounds. Nutritional factors that contribute to the development of pressure ulcers include obesity, being underweight, inadequate food intake, protein deficiency, anemia, hyperglycemia, dehydration, or atherosclerosis.

How to Recognize and Prevent Pressure Ulcers
The four stages of pressure ulcers are:

Stage 1: A pressure ulcer begins with a reddened or purple area of unbroken skin. The skin will remain red for more than 30 minutes after all pressure is removed. Normally, skin will turn white after it has been gently pressed. This is called blanching. On an area that is beginning to form a pressure ulcer, the reddened area of the skin does not blanch. The area may feel warmer than the surrounding skin. For dark-skinned people, this area may be darker than normal. Although the symptoms at this stage may appear insignificant, if left untreated they will quickly progress to those in Stage 2.

Stage 2: The pressure ulcer appears as a raw area of the skin or open cracks in the skin. A small amount of fluid may ooze from the wound.

Stage 3: A crater forms in the tissue, and a significant amount of fluid drains from the area. There is a higher danger of infection.

Stage 4: The wound deepens, reaching into muscle, tendon, or bone, accompanied by substantial fluid drainage. At this stage, pressure ulcers pose a serious threat to the person's health, and may require hospitalization or surgery.

If you see a pressure ulcer at any of the four stages,

alert your physician or home care nurse immediately. Describe the exact location, size (in inches), and condition of the affected area. Pressure ulcers are painful and difficult to treat. The best treatment is prevention. Most pressure ulcers can be prevented.

- Check the skin daily. Bath time is the best time to examine the skin and pressure points with minimum discomfort. Check each pressure point.

- Follow up on complaints about pain, burning, or tingling in the skin. Those sensations may indicate the presence of a pressure ulcer.

- Keep the skin clean and dry. Change moisture-absorbing pads and briefs frequently.

- Never use alkaline soaps or acid deodorants. Use super-fatted soaps or emollients.

- Use soap sparingly; be gentle when bathing in order to maintain skin health.

- Avoid using hot water on the skin.

- Do not let the person sit or lie directly on a pressure ulcer. Absence of pressure is necessary for recovery.

- To help promote circulation, ask the person to wiggle her toes and flex her arms and legs often.

- If the person is unable to move herself, you must reposition her every 2 hours. This is very important in preventing pressure ulcers. A turning chart kept near the bed can be used to chart times and bed positions for each 24 hour period. You can use a clock face to show the time for the next 2-hour position change.

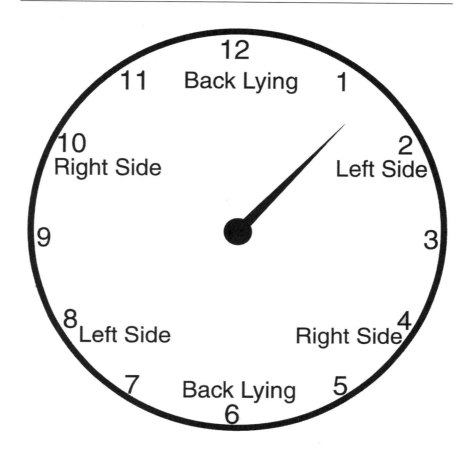

🌿 Never use a heat lamp.

🌿 Do not massage pressure points or reddened areas.

🌿 Make sure splints or braces are fitted and adjusted properly.

🌿 Keep clothing loose and change clothing often.

🌿 Bed sheets should be clean, dry, and free of wrinkles. Wrinkles can cause unnecessary pressure on the skin.

- ❧ Avoid using plastic sheets. Plastic sheets retain urine and body heat, which can cause skin breakdown.

- ❧ Remove the bedpan within 5 minutes after the person has finished using it.

- ❧ Provide a well-balanced, nutritious diet. Encourage the person to drink plenty of fluids.

- ❧ Products are available that help to relieve or reduce pressure on the skin and prevent pressure ulcers. Your doctor, nurse, or home medical supplier can help you select an appropriate product.

- ❧ Improper treatment can make a pressure ulcer worse. Never attempt to treat a pressure ulcer yourself without first consulting trained medical personnel.

Active and Passive Range of Motion Exercises

It is important to continue to exercise the joints and muscles of the body during illness, when normal physical activity may be limited. If joints do not move regularly through their natural range of motion, the surrounding muscles weaken and the joints stiffen, resulting in a condition known as contracture. Your doctor may prohibit exercises for some conditions such as blood clots, fractures, or arthritis. Unless the doctor prohibits exercises, range of motion exercises should be encouraged daily.

Range of motion (ROM) exercises are designed to move muscles and joints through their complete range of motion, helping to maintain strength and flexibility and to increase circulation. Passive ROM exercises require the assistance of another person to help move the person's limbs and body parts. To help move a person safely through a series of passive range of motion exercises, you must first receive instruction on how to perform the exercises from a physical therapist or a nurse. Active range of motion exercises can be done by the person independently.

The following are active range of motion exercises:

Neck

🖖 To exercise the neck, move the head downward as close to the chest as is comfortable. Next, straighten the head.

🖖 With the head level, slowly turn the head to the left as far as is comfortable, then back to center. Slowly turn the head to the right as far as is comfortable. Return to center. Repeat several times.

Shoulders

🖖 To exercise the shoulders, sit up with the back straight. Rotate the shoulders forward in a circular motion, then rotate them back in a circular motion.

🖖 Start with the arms at the side of the body, palms facing inward. Raise one arm straight out in front of the body and continue to raise the arm until it is above the head. Then lower the arm to the starting position. Repeat with the other arm.

🖖 Begin with the arms at the side, palms turned inward. Raise one arm out to the side with the elbow slightly bent. Lift the arm until it is above the head. Lower the arm out to the side until it is back to the starting position. Repeat with the other arm.

Elbow

❧ Start with the arms at the side with the palms turned upward. Bending at the elbow, raise your left forearm toward the left shoulder and try to touch the shoulder with your fingertips. Straighten the arm. Repeat with the other arm.

Forearm and Wrist

❧ To exercise the forearm, begin with the hands straight out in front of the body with the palms face down. Turn the hand so that the palm faces up. Then turn the hand so that the palm faces down again. Repeat several times.

❧ With the hands still straight out in front of the body, palms down, exercise the wrists. Bend the hands downward at the wrist, then straighten the hands and bend them back up toward the forearm. Repeat several times.

Hands and Fingers

❧ Exercise the thumb by touching the tip of each finger with the thumb. Repeat on the other hand.

❧ Exercise the thumb and fingers by holding the fingers and thumb close together and then spreading the fingers and thumb apart. Repeat several times on both hands.

❧ Make the hands into a fist and then release the fist by spreading the thumb and fingers apart. Repeat several times.

Hips

- Start by lying on your back with the body in proper alignment. Keeping the legs straight, exercise the hip by raising and lowering one leg at a time. Repeat several times.

- Keeping the legs straight, slide one leg at a time away from and back towards the body.

Knees

- Start by lying on your back with the body in proper alignment. Exercise one knee at a time. Bend your knee by sliding your foot up until it is next to your other knee. Keep the sole of the foot flat on the bed. Then straighten the leg back to the starting position. Repeat several times.

Ankles, Feet, and Toes

- Flex the foot, bringing the toes up toward the leg and then down away from the leg.

- Raise the foot slightly off the bed and rotate each foot in a circle clockwise and then counterclockwise.

- Exercise the toes by curling the toes and then straightening them. Spread the toes apart and then bring the toes together. Repeat several times.

Personal Hygiene

Mouth Care

- Collect the supplies you will need, including a towel, toothpaste, a toothbrush, a glass of water, a moistened face cloth, a small plastic basin or bowl, and disposable gloves.

🍂 Wash your hands and put on the gloves.

🍂 Encourage the person to clean his own teeth each morning, night, and after meals.

🍂 If the person cannot brush his own teeth, bring him to an upright sitting position.

🍂 Position the towel under the chin and over the chest.

🍂 Apply toothpaste and wet the toothbrush.

🍂 Carefully brush the upper and lower teeth, including the top, front and back sections of each tooth. Brush the tongue.

🍂 When you are finished, ask the person to rinse his mouth with water, spitting afterwards into the basin or bowl. Repeat rinsing until the mouth is clean. Have him rinse with mouthwash if he wishes.

🍂 Wipe the mouth with a moistened face cloth.

🍂 Reposition the person in bed.

🍂 Clean up, and store the supplies.

🍂 Remove the gloves and wash your hands.

How to Clean Dentures

🍂 Dentures should be cleaned at least twice a day and after each meal.

🍂 Gather the equipment you will need, including a soft toothbrush or foam toothette, regular toothpaste, denture toothpaste, a denture cup, a drinking glass for rinsing, a container for used rinse water, paper towels or washcloth, and disposable gloves.

❧ Wash your hands and put on gloves.

❧ Ask the person to remove his or her dentures and place them into the denture cup.

❧ If the person needs assistance, grasp the upper denture and pull it slightly downward to break the suction before gently removing it.

Remove the bottom denture by grasping it and pulling up and then out.

Place the dentures directly into the denture cup.

❧ Place a paper or cloth face towel in the sink to prevent breakage. Dentures can shatter if they are dropped even a short distance.

❧ Rinse the dentures under warm water. Hot water can warp dentures.

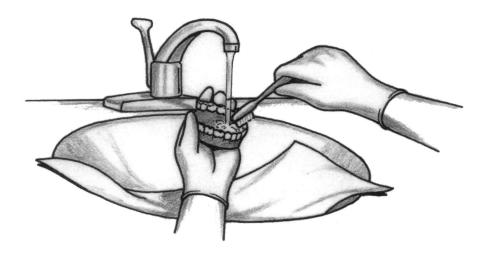

❧ Brush every surface of the dentures using a denture brush. At least once a day, soak the dentures in water with denture cleaning tablets for a more thorough cleaning. Overnight is a good time to soak the dentures.

❧ Clean the person's mouth and stimulate the gums by gently brushing them with a very soft toothbrush. Apply a small amount of toothpaste and wet the toothbrush or use a foam toothette. Rinse the person's mouth with water and use mouthwash if desired.

❧ Return the wet dentures to the person in the denture cup.

❧ If the person needs assistance, return the upper denture to the mouth by holding the denture in one hand and raising the upper lip with the other. Insert the denture and gently press upward on the denture to make sure it is in place. Hold the lower denture in one hand and lower the bottom lip with the other. Insert the denture and gently press downward to bring it into place.

❧ Rinse and dry the denture cup. Remove the gloves and wash your hands.

Shaving

❧ Gather the supplies you will need: disposable gloves, razor, shaving cream or gel, towel, warm moist washcloth, basin of warm water and after shave lotion (optional).

❧ If possible, raise the bed to a comfortable working height.

❧ Move the person into an upright or sitting position.

❧ Wash your hands and put on the gloves. If the person you are caring for wears dentures, make sure that they are in place. Position a towel underneath the chin and across the chest.

❧ If you are going to use a blade razor, place a warm washcloth on the person's face for a few moments to soften the beard.

❧ Apply shaving cream and lather the area to be shaved.

❧ Start in front of one ear. Hold the skin taut by pressing at the cheek and pulling the skin toward the ear.

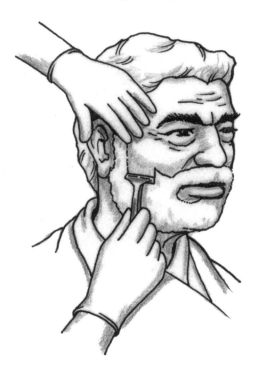

Take short, even strokes in the direction the hair grows. Shave the neck by bringing the razor toward the chin. Rinse the razor between strokes in a basin of warm water.

ﻉ Rinse the face with a warm washcloth. Pat dry with a towel. Apply after shave lotion if desired.

ﻉ Be careful not to irritate sensitive areas. If the skin has been nicked, hold a tissue or gauze pad directly over the spot, applying slight pressure for a few moments.

ﻉ Clean, rinse, dry, and store the supplies.

ﻉ Remove the gloves and wash your hands.

ﻉ Never use an electric razor if a person is receiving oxygen because of the potential for sparks that could ignite a fire.

Nail Care

ﻉ Consult with a podiatrist for special cases such as thick nails, poor circulation, or diabetes. Special precautions need to be taken when cutting the nails of a diabetic. The podiatrist can cut the nails or give instruction.

ﻉ Gather the necessary supplies: soap, water, basin, nail brush, towel, small scissors or clippers, and an emery board or nail file.

ﻉ Wash your hands.

ﻉ The best time to trim nails is after a bath or after a warm foot or hand soak. The nails are less hard and brittle after soaking.

- Brush the nails with a nail brush, cleaning under the nails. Rinse and dry the nails and hands.

- When clipping the nails, make a straight cut for toenails and a curved cut for fingernails. Work over a paper or cloth towel to make cleanup easier.

- Use the nail file or emery board to smooth the edges of the nails.

- Clean and store the equipment. Wash your hands.

How to Shampoo the Hair in Bed

- Gather the supplies you will need, including a waterproof sheet, shampoo, conditioner, towels, plastic shampoo tray, comb and brush, a large pitcher for warm water, and a water collection bucket.

- Tell the person what you plan to do.

- Remove the person's hearing aids and/or eyeglasses.

- Wash your hands.

- If possible, position the bed to a convenient height.

- Place a waterproof sheet underneath the person's head and shoulders.

- Position the person so that his head is near the bed's edge.

- Place the shampoo tray underneath his head. Position the drain tube into the water collection bucket.

- Gently wet the hair using a large pitcher of warm water (about 100 degrees).

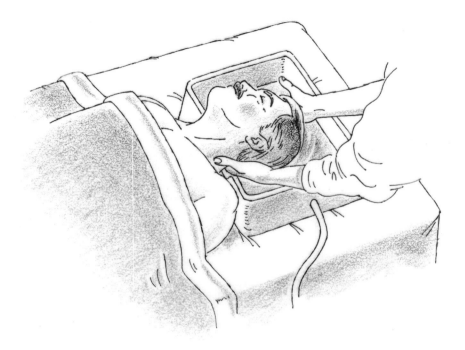

🌿 Apply a small amount of shampoo into the wet hair, lathering well and massaging the scalp gently.

🌿 Rinse the hair thoroughly.

🌿 Use conditioner if desired. Rinse thoroughly.

🌿 Remove the shampoo tray from the bed.

🌿 Wrap the hair with a large towel.

🌿 If you use a hair dryer, adjust the temperature to the coolest setting and dry the hair.

🌿 Clean and store the equipment and wash your hands.

How to Give a Bed Bath

For most people, bathing provides a sense of well being and relaxation as it cleanses the skin, refreshes the spirit, and stimulates circulation. Daily bathing is not advisable in some situations. Check with the doctor or nurse about how often to give a bath or shower. If a person is incontinent or perspires heavily, daily bathing is necessary.

- Bath time is the best time to check for bedsores, swelling, rashes, or other unusual skin changes.
- Gather the supplies that you will need: disposable gloves, mild soap, wash cloths, towels and bath towels, wash basin, nail brush, and clean clothes.
- The room should be warm. Close the windows to avoid a draft.
- Offer the bedpan or urinal to the person before beginning the bed bath.
- Wash your hands.
- Use good body mechanics: stand with your feet apart, your knees bent, and your back straight.
- Always tell the person what you plan to do, step by step.
- Allow the person to help as much as possible.
- Put on disposable gloves.
- Remove the person's clothes. Remove heavy blankets or bedspreads. Uncover only the area you want to wash, leaving the rest of the body covered with top sheet, a bath towel, or light blanket.

- Start with the cleanest areas of the body, such as the face, chest, and arms. Wash progressively to the most soiled areas, such as feet, buttocks, and rectal area. Change the water frequently as it becomes dirty or cool.

- Use one washcloth for soap and one for rinsing. Washcloths should be wet, but not dripping.

- Using only clean water, start by washing the eyes. Wipe from the inner corner to the outer corner of the eye. Use the opposite end of the washcloth for the second eye.

- Wash the face using soap. Wash the ears and neck. Rinse thoroughly and pat dry.

- Place a bath towel underneath the arm and hand to keep the bed dry. Support the arm by holding it beneath the elbow. Wash the arm upward from the wrist to the shoulder to stimulate circulation. Rinse and pat dry. Wash under the arm. Place the hand in a small basin of warm water and let it soak for a minute. Wash the hand, including the areas between the fingers. Check the nails. Use a nail brush to clean under the nails. Repeat the procedure for the other hand and arm.

- Wash the chest. For females, the area under the breasts should be washed as well.

- Wash the stomach and abdomen.

- Ask the person to bend his or her knee. Support the leg beneath the knee as you wash the leg, moving

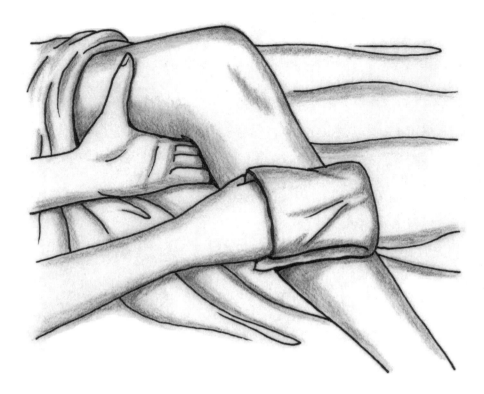

from ankle to upper thigh to stimulate circulation. Rinse. Soak the foot in a basin of water before washing. Support the foot by holding at the heel or ankle. Wash the foot, paying attention to the areas between the toes. Check the nails. Clean with a nail brush if necessary. Repeat the procedure for the other leg and foot.

🌿 Change the water in the basin before continuing with the bath.

❦ Turn the person on his or her side and place a large bath towel lengthwise along the back and the buttocks. Starting at the neck, use long strokes to wash the back from the neck down to and including the buttocks. Rinse well and pat dry.

❦ Place a towel up against the buttocks and turn the person onto his or her back so that the buttocks are on the towel. If at all possible, let the person wash his or her own genital and anal areas. You can help by preparing washcloths and having the towel ready.

❦ If you must wash the genital area, begin by telling the person what you plan to do.

❦ If the male is uncircumcised, retract the foreskin. Wash, rinse, and pat dry the penis. Return the foreskin to its original position. Gently wash, rinse, and pat dry the scrotum.

❦ For females, help her to flex her knees and spread her legs if able. Gently wash the genitals from the front downwards toward the rectum, rinsing after each stroke. Repeat until the area is clean. Pat dry thoroughly with a towel.

❦ Prepare to wash the rectal area by positioning the person onto his or her side with knees bent. Lift the upper buttock with one hand. With the other hand, clean the area with soap and water from the vagina or scrotum to the anus using a single gentle stroke. Rinse between each stroke, and repeat the process using a clean section of the washcloth until the area is clean. Pat dry thoroughly.

🍃 PeriWash, an antibacterial cleanser for the genital area, can be used to help reduce bacteria.

🍃 Dress the person in clean clothes. Comb, brush, or wash the hair.

🍃 Change the bed linens. Place soiled linen and towels in the laundry container.

🍃 Discard disposable items. Clean and store other equipment.

🍃 Remove the gloves and wash your hands.

How to Make an Occupied Bed

It may be necessary to make a bed with the person in it if he or she is unable to get out of bed.

Bed linens must be changed often, for comfort and to reduce the possibility of infection. It's important that the bed be made free of wrinkles to prevent pressure sores from developing.

🍃 If you are using a hospital bed, raise the bed to the level of your elbows and lower the knee and head sections until the bed is flat.

🍃 The procedure will vary slightly if you use a draw sheet or additional bed pads.

🍃 Loosen the sheets and blankets around the entire bed.

🍃 Remove all the covers, except for the top sheet or a cotton blanket to keep the person warm.

🍃 Roll the person to the far side of the bed. He should be on his side, facing away from you. If the bed has side rails, raise the rail on the far side of the bed. If not, position the bed against a wall or secure the person in the bed with pillows.

🕭 Remove the head pillow.

🕭 Place the clean linen within easy reach.

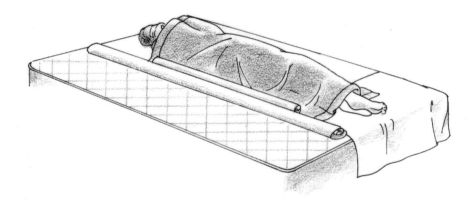

🕭 Fold or roll any bed pad or draw sheet toward the person and tuck it against the person's back. Roll or fold the bottom sheet lengthwise up against the person's back. Your side of the bed should now be stripped down to the mattress or mattress pad and ready for clean linens.

🕭 If you are using a flat sheet, take the sheet and fold it in half lengthwise.

🕭 Place the folded edge of the sheet lengthwise up against the body from the top to the bottom of the bed.

🕭 Fold or roll the top half of the clean flat sheet (the portion that will go on the other side of the bed) and tuck it under the person's back. The half of the bed you are working on should now have the bottom sheet ready to be tucked into the mattress. Tuck the sheet in at the head of the bed, along the side, and at the foot of the bed. If you need additional bed pads or a draw sheet, follow the same procedure.

🌾 When using a fitted sheet, place the fitted corner on the top and bottom corners of the side of the bed near you. Then smooth the sheet at the center and push the sheet against the person's body.

🌾 You are now ready to move the person over to the clean side of the bed. Roll him gently onto his back and over the bunched linens in the middle of the bed. If there are no side rails, stabilize the person with pillows so that he or she does not roll any further.

🌾 Move to the "dirty" side of the bed. Remove the soiled linens and place them in the laundry bag. The bed should be stripped to the mattress or mattress pad on that side of the bed. Pull the clean sheet from the middle of the bed and pull it firmly to make a tight, wrinkle-free bed, tucking it in at the head, along the side, and at the foot of the bed. Pull any additional pads or draw sheet from the center, and tuck anything that hangs over the edge of the bed under the mattress.

🌾 Change the pillow case.

🌾 Change the top sheet. Be sure to leave room for the feet to move freely when you tuck it in at the foot of the bed. Spread a blanket over the top sheet. Sometimes the weight of the blankets on the person's body will cause pain or discomfort. A blanket support can help. The blanket support sits on the bed and holds the blanket and sheet away from the person's body.

❧ Reposition the person comfortably in the bed.

How to Put on Elasticized Stockings

Elasticized stockings, sometimes called TEDs, are used to improve circulation and to prevent swelling or formation of blood clots in the legs. They come in a variety of sizes and lengths. The legs are measured to determine the proper stocking length.

❧ Elasticized stockings should be changed daily after bathing.

❧ Stockings should be removed and put on again every 8 hours, to check the color and warmth of the feet and toes. When putting elastic stockings on, use this procedure:

- Wash your hands.
- Tell the person what you plan to do.
- With the person lying down, expose one leg at a time.
- Make sure the legs are clean and dry.
- Gather the stocking down to the heel.
- Pull the stocking over the person's foot and heel. Check that the heel is properly placed in the heel of the stocking.

- Continue to pull the stocking upward over the leg. When you have finished, the stocking should be smooth, with no wrinkles.

- Repeat the procedure for the other leg.

- Make sure that the person is comfortable.

- Wash your hands.

Elimination

Many wonderful new products are now available that are helpful for elimination, such as female urinals (including urinals for women in wheelchairs), bedpans that are flatter, wider and more comfortable, and protective briefs that are noiseless, control odors and are capable of holding large amounts of fluid without feeling wet. Check the resources section under "Incontinence" for the names of suppliers of these new products.

How to Use a Bedpan

Using a bedpan is often a source of shame or embarrassment. Remember that preserving the person's dignity is an important part of caregiving.

- Gather supplies: disposable gloves, bedpan, toilet paper, and two moistened washcloths, (optional supplies: oil, disposable wipes, talcum powder, bell).

- Allow for privacy during bedpan use.

- Wash your hands.

- Always wear gloves when you are helping someone use a bedpan.

- A cold bedpan is uncomfortable. Run warm water over the bedpan immediately before use. Dry the pan thoroughly and apply talcum powder to reduce friction.

- Place a tissue or a little water or oil on the bottom of the pan before use to make cleaning easier.

- The bed should be in a flat position.

- Pull the lower garment below the knees and the upper garment above the waist.

- If the person can assist you, ask him to bend his knees and press his heels against the bed while raising his hips. Slide your hand under the lower part of the back, and gently lift the hips at the same time.

- Slide the bedpan under the hips; the buttocks should rest on the rounded shelf of the bedpan. The narrow end of the bedpan should point toward the foot of the bed.

- If the person cannot raise his hips, turn him onto his side with his back facing you. Position the bedpan against the buttocks. Then, roll him back over the bedpan, checking to be sure the pan is in the proper position. (See illustration, p. 91)

- Elevate the head of the bed, or assist the person into a semi-sitting position using pillows for support. For added privacy, adjust the position of the sheet to cover the person.

- Place toilet paper within reach.

- Leave a moist washcloth nearby for cleaning.

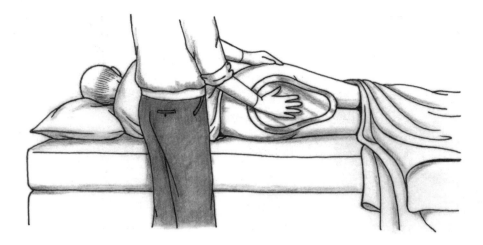

- When he is comfortable, leave the room.

- Keep a bell next to the bed so he can alert you when he is finished.

- Always remove the bedpan as soon as the person is finished using it. A bedpan left in place for more than 15 minutes can cause the first stages of skin breakdown, leading to a pressure ulcer.

- Remove the bedpan by lowering the bed or removing the pillows so that he is lying on his back. Have him raise his hips by flexing his knees and placing his feet flat on the bed. You can help raise the hips by placing one hand under the small of the back and lifting. Gently slide the bedpan from underneath with your other hand.

- Hand him the toilet paper and allow him to clean

himself if possible. Discard the used paper in the bed-pan. Follow with a moistened washcloth, so he can wash the rectal area. Use a second washcloth for washing the hands.

- If he needs help to clean himself, assist him onto his side, with his knees bent. Lift his upper buttock with one hand. With your other hand, clean the area from the scrotum to the anus with soap and water using a single gentle stroke. Clean from the vagina to the anus for females. Rinse between each stroke, and repeat the process using a clean section of the wash-cloth each time until the area is clean. Disposable wipes can be helpful. Pat dry thoroughly.

- Reposition him until he is comfortable in the bed.

- Empty the bedpan contents into the toilet, and clean the bedpan using warm, soapy water and a toilet brush. Rinse and dry.

- Remove and discard the disposable gloves. Wash your hands.

How to Use a Male Urinal

- Wash your hands and put on disposable gloves.

- Place the urinal between the legs, low enough so that the penis can naturally be inserted into the urinal. Provide assistance if necessary.

- Leave him alone in the room if possible. When he lets you know that he is finished, remove and empty the urinal, measuring if necessary.

🕊 Clean the urinal with warm soapy water. Rinse with disinfectant or water and dry.

🕊 Wash his hands, or provide him with a moistened washcloth.

🕊 Remove and discard the gloves and wash your hands.

Urinary Incontinence

Urinary incontinence is an involuntary loss of urine in sufficient amounts or frequency to cause social and/or health problems.

Normal urination during daytime hours occurs no more than once every 2 hours. Going to the bathroom 1-2 times during the night is considered normal.

The four types of urinary incontinence are stress, urge, overflow, and functional.

1. Stress incontinence occurs during coughing, laughing, sneezing, or physical activities such as lifting. Weak pelvic floor muscles are a common cause of stress incontinence.

2. Urge incontinence involves sudden loss of urine because of the urge to urinate. The person is unable to reach the bathroom in time. Urge incontinence is often seen in people who have diabetes, stroke, dementia, Parkinson's or multiple sclerosis.

3. Overflow incontinence involves frequent leakage of small amounts of urine. The bladder is overextended as a result of loss of bladder muscle tone or an outlet obstruction.

4. Functional incontinence occurs when the bladder and urinary tract are healthy but the person is still unable

or unwilling to use a toilet. Causes can include difficulty moving, pain, clothing, and psychological factors.

Causes of Urinary Incontinence

Urinary incontinence may be caused by diverticula, kidney or bladder stones, chronic immobility, diabetes, enlarged prostate, hormonal imbalance, physical disabilities, mental confusion, or neurological disorders such as multiple sclerosis. Vaginal infection or urinary infection may also cause urinary incontinence. Diuretic substances, such as certain drugs, alcohol, and caffeine can affect bladder function. Some tranquilizers and sedatives may make the person so drowsy that he or she may sleep through the need to eliminate. If the problem is caused by medications, your doctor may be able to improve the situation by changing dosage amounts or administration times. Do not change the timing or dosage of any medication unless you are specifically directed to do so by the physician.

The cause of urinary incontinence, especially if it comes on quickly, should always be evaluated by the doctor. Do not assume that it is a result of old age or confusion. A sudden onset of urinary incontinence can often be corrected.

General Guidelines When Caring for Someone with Incontinence

- Avoid tight fitting clothes, which can produce pressure on the bladder.
- Provide clothing that can be easily removed.
- Avoid coffee, tea, alcohol, chocolate, carbonated bev-

erages, spicy foods, tomatoes, and citrus, which can irritate the bladder and cause frequent urination.

๏ Avoid evening fluids; however, total fluid intake should not be restricted. Continue to encourage the person to drink 6-8 cups of water daily.

๏ Keep the skin of an incontinent person clean and dry. Urine left on the skin can cause pressure ulcers and infection.

๏ Be alert for skin dryness or breakdown, rash, or infection. Inspect the person's skin frequently, and make sure to report any changes immediately to the doctor or home care nurse.

๏ Apply hypoallergenic creams or oils to protect the skin.

๏ Allow privacy when the person is urinating.

๏ Keep hallways free of clutter and make the bathroom as accessible as possible.

Treating Urinary Incontinence

You may be asked to keep a bladder urination record for three days to see if there is any pattern. This record helps to identify the type of incontinence and determine the treatment plan. Recorded information usually includes the times urination occurs, the amount, presence of urge, activities associated with the loss, daily number of pad changes, fluid intake, and intake of any dietary irritants.

๏ After the cause of urinary incontinence has been medically established, bladder training, medications, surgery, or exercises may be prescribed to improve or correct the situation.

🕊 Urge incontinence and stress incontinence can be helped with bladder training. Prompted voiding (urinating at predetermined times based on the bladder urination record) is a technique used to retrain the bladder.

🕊 Pelvic muscle exercises called Kegel exercises are prescribed for stress incontinence, to strengthen weak muscles around the bladder.

🕊 For urge incontinence, electrical stimulation may be used along with medications.

🕊 Functional incontinence may require an assessment by a physical therapist, use of an assistive walking device such as a walker or cane, and proper shoes, exercise, and foot care.

Fecal Incontinence

Fecal incontinence may be caused by weakness of the anal sphincter, certain nervous system disorders, immobility, or mental confusion.

🕊 Providing a high-fiber diet and adequate water intake is important in maintaining bowel health.

🕊 Bowel training (offering the toilet or bedpan at regularly scheduled times) may improve continence. The best time for many people is after each meal.

🕊 Provide privacy and make sure that the person is comfortable.

❧ Give the person enough time to defecate. Do not give the impression that you want him to finish in a hurry. A bell or other device near the bed will allow him to call you when he is finished.

❧ Clean the incontinent person thoroughly after each bowel movement to prevent development of pressure ulcers and infections.

Adult Briefs

Adult briefs keep an incontinent person dry, reduce odor, lessen the chance of urinary infections and pressure sores, and help prevent embarrassment if there is an accident. Adult briefs come in a variety of sizes and styles, from insert pads for specially designed reusable briefs to wraparound disposable briefs fastened with tabs.

❧ Follow the manufacturer's instructions for a proper fit. It is important that the briefs fit well.

❧ Briefs should be checked and changed every 2 hours. Many are equipped with a strip that changes color when they need to be changed.

❧ Adult briefs are available at the local home medical supply store, large pharmacies, and grocery stores.

Using Urinary ("Foley") Catheters

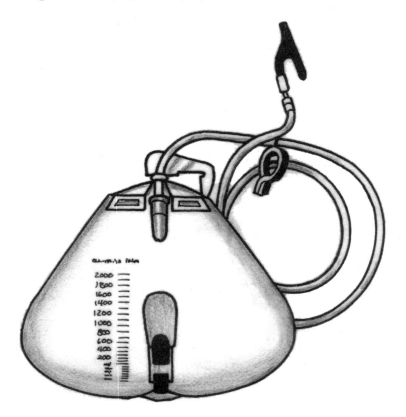

An indwelling urinary catheter allows for constant urine drainage. Catheters are used after surgery or to manage urinary incontinence. The catheter is inserted through the urethra into the bladder by a nurse and held in place by a balloon that is inflated once it is in the bladder. This prevents the catheter from slipping out of the bladder.

❦ The inside of the catheter and drainage system are sterile. Do not insert anything into the catheter tubing or collection bag. When disconnecting the system, be careful not to let the disconnected tubing touch anything. Cap it or reconnect it immediately.

❧ The drainage bag should always be located lower than the person's bladder to prevent backflow.

❧ Check the catheter often to make sure that there are no folds or kinks in the catheter or tubing. Arrange the drainage tubing in a coil and tape it to the lower bed sheet to prevent drainage problems.

❧ Never attach the drainage bag or tubing to a movable part of the bed such as the side rails. Raising and lowering the bed rails might dislodge the catheter. Attach the collection bag to the bed frame.

❧ Never pull on the catheter.

❧ Check the color, odor, amount, and character of the urine. Report anything unusual to the doctor or home care nurse immediately.

❧ Immediately report any signs of urine leakage around the catheter to the nurse.

❧ If the person has pain, burning, irritation, a full feeling in the bladder, or an ongoing urge to urinate, report it to the doctor or nurse immediately.

How to Clean a Urinary Catheter

People using indwelling catheters are at risk for developing urinary tract infection. To prevent infection, it is essential to keep the catheter insertion area clean.

❧ Assemble the supplies you will need: disposable

gloves, a washcloth and soap and warm water, anti-septic wipes, a towel or bed protector, and a plastic bag for waste.

🖐 Wash your hands and put on disposable gloves.

🖐 Tell the person what you plan to do.

🖐 If possible, raise the bed to a comfortable working height.

🖐 Place a towel or bed protector under the buttocks. Position the person on his or her back.

🖐 Expose only the area where the catheter enters the body.

🖐 Using soap and warm water, wash the area where the catheter enters the body and several inches along the catheter. For females, separate the labia and wash the area from front to back. For males, clean the head of the penis.

🖐 Check for anything abnormal such as leakage, skin breakdown, bleeding, or signs of infection. Report any of these to the doctor or home care nurse immediately.

🖐 Using antiseptic wipes, wipe the catheter tube. Start near the insertion site and continue wiping down to the place where the catheter connects to the drainage tubing, being careful not to dislodge or disconnect the catheter.

🖐 Remove the bed protector from underneath the person.

🖐 Make sure the catheter is in place and the tubing

secure. Tubing should not be below the collection bag.

🌿 Check the level of urine in the collection bag and empty if necessary.

🌿 Remove the gloves and discard them into the plastic bag.

How to Empty the Collection Bag

🌿 Gather the equipment you will need: disposable gloves, alcohol wipes, measuring device (a marked container into which you will drain the contents of the collection bag), and a towel, paper towels, or newspaper.

🌿 Wash your hands and put on the gloves.

🌿 Tell the person what you plan to do.

🌿 Place a towel, paper towels, or newspaper on the floor below the collection bag. Place the container on the towel, directly under the spout at the bottom of the collection bag.

🌿 Open the drain spout and allow the urine to flow into the container. Do not allow the catheter tube to touch the container.

🌿 When the urine has drained, close the drain and wipe it with an alcohol wipe. Replace the drain into the holder on the collection bag.

🌿 Measure and record urine output. Observe the urine for any changes in color, character or sediment. Report these changes to the doctor or nurse immediately. Empty the urine into the toilet and flush. Wash and rinse the container.

🕊 Remove the gloves and wash your hands.

How to Connect the Leg Bag

🕊 A leg bag allows for greater mobility than the bedside collection bag, but it needs to be emptied more often.

🕊 Gather the equipment you will need: disposable gloves, leg bag, alcohol wipes, and paper towels.

🕊 Wash your hands and put on the gloves.

🕊 Tell the person what you plan to do.

🕊 Place a paper towel underneath the catheter connection area.

🕊 Disinfect the catheter connection area with an alcohol wipe.

🕊 Disconnect the catheter from the tubing. Wipe the end of the catheter with an alcohol wipe. Remove the cap from the end of the leg bag and connect the leg bag to the catheter. Wipe the end of the bedside drainage bag tubing with an alcohol wipe. Place a cap on the end of the tube to keep the drainage system closed.

🕊 Attach the leg straps and bag to the person's leg. Check to make sure that the part marked "top of bag" is in the correct position, and that the straps are smooth and not too tight. Check the tubing for folds or kinks.

❧ Empty and measure the urine from the bedside collection bag.

❧ Remove the gloves and wash your hands.

How to Clear a Blocked Catheter

If urine hasn't drained for 2 hours even though the person has been drinking fluids, the catheter may be blocked. Other signs of a blocked catheter include feeling pressure in the lower abdomen or the urge to urinate.

❧ Straighten any kinks in the catheter tubing.

❧ Check the position of the collection bag. It should be lower than the level of the bladder. Adjust the position if necessary.

❧ Sometimes the catheter moves into a position against the bladder wall and urine cannot flow through the catheter. Changing the person's body position may help to restore the flow of urine.

❧ Catheter irrigation can correct catheter blockage. Do not attempt to irrigate the catheter until you have been trained by a nurse.

❧ Never remove the catheter unless instructed to do so by the doctor or nurse.

Applying and Using a Condom Catheter

Condom catheters, when left on for long periods of time, may cause skin breakdown. This can be prevented by using the condom catheter during the night time only. A urinal is used during the day. Some condom catheters are self-adhesive; others come with skin preparation supplies and tape.

- Collect the materials you will need: self-adhesive condom catheter or condom catheter with skin prep supplies, collection bag with tubing, soap, washcloth, and towel.

- Wash your hands.

- Provide privacy.

- The person should be lying on his back.

- Put on gloves.

- Wash the penis with soap and water, using a wash-cloth. If the male is uncircumcised, retract the foreskin. Wash, rinse, and pat dry the penis. Return the foreskin to its original position. Gently wash, rinse, and pat dry the scrotum. You may need to trim the hair at the base of the penis to keep it from sticking to the tape.

- Attach the collection bag to the leg or the bed frame.

- If using a self-adhesive condom catheter, apply a protective coating such as skin prep to the skin of the penis before applying the condom. Follow the manufacturer's instructions for non-adhesive catheters which come with skin preparation supplies. When using tape, avoid overlapping or stretching the tape, which can cut off circulation.

- Roll the edges of the condom catheter toward the tip, in the same way you would roll up a sock.

- Place the catheter sheath on the end of the penis,

leaving about 1/2" of space between the tip of the penis and the connector tip.

🌿 Gently stretch the penis as you unroll the condom. When the condom is unrolled, gently press it against the penis so that it sticks to the tape or, if self-adhesive, sticks to the penis.

🌿 Connect one end of the tubing to the connector tip and other other end to the collection bag.

🌿 Check that the tip of the catheter is straight and that the tubing is relaxed and free of kinks.

🌿 Discard used supplies.

🌿 Remove and discard the gloves.

🌿 Wash your hands.

🌿 Empty the collection bag every 3-4 hours. Do not let it fill to the top.

🌿 Wash the collection bag twice a day with soap and water. Rinse with a solution of 1 part vinegar to 7 parts water.

🌿 Remove the condom catheter by first disconnecting the drainage tube. Keep the top of the drainage tube clean; you can place it in a clean container. Roll the condom catheter and any tape toward the head of the penis. Use a skin prep adhesive remover to help with tape removal.

🌿 Change the condom catheter every 24 hours. Thoroughly wash and dry the penis between changes.

🌿 Check the penis every 2 hours for color changes or

swelling. Report any changes to the nurse or doctor, including any pain or burning during urination or changes in the color or smell of the urine.

How to Give a Prepackaged Enema

Do not administer the enema if the person has abdominal pain, nausea or is vomiting.

🌿 Gather disposable gloves, the prepackaged enema, a protective pad, a bedpan (if necessary), toilet paper, lubrication jelly, water, washcloth, soap, and towel.

🌿 Warm the enema by placing the bottle in a pan of warm water. Warm only to body temperature.

🌿 Wash your hands and put on the gloves.

🌿 Tell the person what you plan to do.

🌿 Provide privacy.

🌿 Place the protective pad underneath the buttocks. The person should be lying on his or her side, with knees bent and the covers turned back to expose only the buttocks.

🌿 Remove the cover from the tip of the enema. Apply some extra lubricant to the tip of the enema to ease insertion.

🌿 Separate the buttocks by raising the top buttock. Ask the person to exhale as you insert the pointed tip of the enema tube into the rectum at least 2 inches. Slowly squeeze the bottle to send the solution into the rectum in an even flow. Stop if you feel resistance or if the person complains of pain or cramping. Resume when the cramping stops.

⚘ When all of the solution has flowed into the rectum, hold the buttocks together while you remove the enema tip. The person may feel an urge to empty the bowel. Encourage him or her to hold the solution for the length of time recommended on the enema instructions.

⚘ Assist the person to the toilet (or with a bedpan) if necessary.

⚘ Be sure that toilet paper is within reach, and leave the room if possible.

⚘ When you return, assist with the cleanup if necessary.

⚘ Return the person to a comfortable position, leaving the protective pad in place until you are sure that the effects of the enema are complete.

⚘ If necessary, record the results of the enema for the physician.

⚘ Remove the gloves and wash your hands.

How to Administer a Rectal Suppository

Suppositories are usually wrapped in foil and kept in the refrigerator. Once the suppository has been inserted into the rectum, it will melt in 5 to 10 minutes. Make sure the person waits at least that long before trying to have a bowel movement.

⚘ Gather the supplies: disposable gloves, suppository, water-soluble lubricant, and a protective pad or paper towels.

🍂 Wash your hands and put on the gloves.

🍂 Tell the person what you plan to do.

🍂 Place the protective pad or towel underneath the person's buttocks.

🍂 The person should be lying on his or her side with knees bent and the covers turned back to expose only the buttocks. Open the foil-wrapped suppository.

🍂 Lubricate the tip of the suppository and your gloved index finger with the water-soluble lubricant.

🍂 With the other hand, lift the top buttock.

🍂 Gently insert the suppository into the rectum. Push it past the sphincter muscles of the rectum and along the lining of the rectum as far as your index finger allows—about 3 inches. Try not to insert the suppository into feces. The suppository is most effective next to the lining of the colon.

🍂 Ask the person to hold the suppository for 10-20 minutes.

🍂 Remove the gloves and wash your hands.

🍂 After 10-20 minutes, he or she may feel an urge to have a bowel movement. Assist the person to the toilet, or provide a bedpan if necessary.

Vital Signs

Vital signs provide valuable information on how the body is functioning by measuring body temperature, pulse, respiratory rates, and blood pressure.

How to Take the Temperature

The three methods for taking the temperature are: rectal, oral, and axillary (under the armpit). The rectal method is the most accurate, the oral method is second in accuracy, and the axillary method is least accurate. If you are in doubt about which method to use, ask your doctor or home care nurse.

Temperature readings will vary slightly depending on which method you use. Normal body temperature varies from person to person. Body temperature also varies slightly at different times of the day.

	Average	Range
Rectal	99.6	98.6-100.6 F
Oral	98.6	97.6-99.6 F
Axillary	97.6	96.6-98.6 F

About Thermometers

- The two most common types of thermometers are digital and glass thermometers.

- Digital thermometers let you know when to read the temperature at the sound of a beep and have a display that shows the numerical temperature.

- The two types of glass thermometers are oral and rectal. An oral thermometer is used to take both oral and axillary temperatures. A rectal thermometer, which has a thicker, rounder end, is used to take rectal temperatures.

- Never use an oral thermometer to take the temperature rectally (or vice versa) for hygienic and safety reasons.

How to Read the Thermometer

❧ The glass thermometer reads temperatures ranging from 94 to 108 degrees. Long and short lines on the side of the thermometer indicate measurements: each long line represents one degree; each short line two-tenths of one degree.

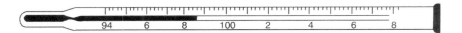

❧ Check the existing thermometer reading before taking the temperature.

❧ Hold the thermometer by the end of its stem at eye level.

❧ Turn the thermometer slowly until you see the silvery column of mercury.

❧ The mercury column should read 96F (35.6C) or lower. If it does not, hold the thermometer firmly and shake the mercury down by snapping your wrist downward until it reads 96F (35.6C) or lower.

❧ Mercury within the thermometer expands and rises as it is heated by the body, giving the temperature reading.

Taking an Oral Temperature

❧ Gather supplies: thermometer, gloves, alcohol wipe or soap and water, and a watch or clock for timing.

❧ Oral thermometers require that the person hold the thermometer in his or her closed mouth for several minutes. Safety is a consideration, because glass thermometers can break. If the person is confused, use another method for taking the temperature.

❧ Certain activities affect oral temperature readings. Wait at least 15 minutes before taking the temperature if the person has just eaten or drunk, smoked, exercised, or bathed.

❧ Wash your hands and put on the gloves.

❧ Check the temperature reading on the thermometer. The mercury column should read 96F (35.6C) or lower. If it does not, hold the thermometer firmly and shake the mercury down by snapping your wrist downward until it reads 96F (35.6C) or lower.

❧ Insert the bulb end of the thermometer under the tongue, slanted toward the side of the mouth. Keep the thermometer under the tongue for a minimum of 3 minutes.

❧ Read the temperature by holding the thermometer at eye level, turning it slowly until you see the silvery column of mercury. Average oral temperature is 98.6F. The normal range is 97.6 - 99.6F (36.5 - 37.5C) If the person's temperature exceeds 101F (38C), report it to the doctor or home care nurse immediately.

🍃 Wipe the thermometer with an alcohol wipe from stem end to bulb end or wash with soap and water. Rinse well.

🍃 Remove the gloves and wash your hands.

🍃 Record the temperature reading if requested by the nurse or doctor.

Taking an Axillary Temperature

🍃 Gather supplies: thermometer, alcohol wipes or soap and water, and a watch or clock for timing.

🍃 Wait 15 minutes after the person has washed or applied deodorant before taking the axillary temperature.

🍃 Remove the clothing from the shoulder and arm. Dry the armpit.

🍃 Check the temperature reading on the thermometer. The mercury column should read 96F (35.6C) or lower. If it does not, hold the thermometer firmly and shake the mercury down by snapping your wrist downward until it reads 96F (35.6C) or lower.

🍃 Place the thermometer with the bulb end in the center of the armpit.

🍃 Bring the arm close to the body and place the forearm over the chest to hold the thermometer in place. Leave in place for ten minutes.

🍃 Read the temperature by holding the thermometer at eye level, turning it slowly, until you see the silvery column of mercury.

- Average axillary temperature is 97.6F (36.5C). The normal range is 96.6 - 98.6F (36 - 37C). If the axillary temperature exceeds 100F (38C), report to the doctor or nurse immediately.

- Wipe the thermometer clean with an alcohol wipe or wash with soap and water. Rinse well.

- Wash your hands.

Taking a Rectal Temperature

- Gather supplies: rectal thermometer, gloves, alcohol wipes or soap and water, and a watch or clock for timing.

- Wash your hands and put on gloves.

- Position the person on his or her left side with knees bent. Move the clothing away from the buttocks and rectal area.

- Check the temperature reading on the thermometer. The mercury column should read 96F (35.6C) or lower. If it does not, hold the thermometer firmly and shake the mercury down by snapping your wrist downward until it reads 96F (35.6C) or lower.

- Place a small quantity of water-soluble lubricant on a tissue and lubricate the tip of the thermometer.

- With one hand, raise the top buttock, and with the other hand gently insert the bulb end of the thermometer into the rectum about 1 to 1 1/2 inches.

- Hold the thermometer in place for 3 to 5 minutes. Do not let go of the thermometer.

❧ Remove the thermometer and wipe it with an alcohol-saturated pad in one stroke from stem to bulb. Discard the pad and wipe again with a new pad if necessary.

❧ Read the temperature. Average rectal temperature is 99.6F (37.5C). The normal range is 98.6 -100.6F (37 - 38.1C). If the rectal temperature exceeds 102F (39C), report it to the doctor or nurse.

❧ Clean the thermometer again by using an alcohol-soaked pad or soap and water. Rinse thoroughly.

❧ Remove and discard the gloves and wash your hands.

How to Take the Pulse

When the heart contracts, it starts the movement of blood through the arteries and this throbbing of the artery as the blood is pushed against the artery walls is the pulse. The pulse rate should be the same as the heart rate. The average adult pulse rate is 60-100 beats per minute.

❧ The most common site for checking the pulse is the radial artery, which you can feel inside the wrist on the thumb side. Other places you can find a pulse are the temples, at each side of the neck, behind the knee, and the top of the foot.

❧ Exercise, pain, fear, and fever can elevate the pulse rate.

❧ Certain medications may elevate or lower pulse rate.

❧ Wait 15 minutes after exercise or activity before taking the pulse.

❧ Wash your hands.

❧ Have the person sit or lie quietly with arms at rest on the chest.

❧ Place the tips of your first two fingers on the person's inner wrist on the thumb side. Feel for the pulse by pressing along the inner wrist, but do not press too hard or it will make it difficult to find and count the pulse.

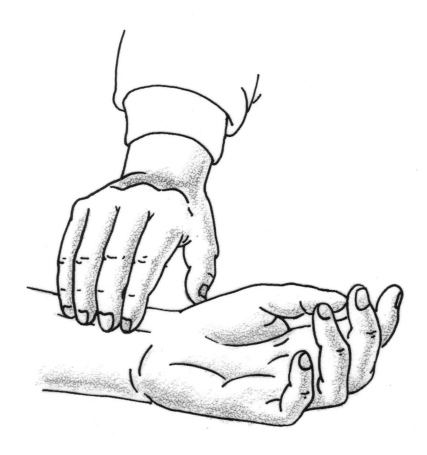

ᴪ Never use your thumb to take the pulse. Your thumb has a pulse of its own which makes it difficult to get an accurate reading.

ᴪ Count pulse beats for 1 full minute. Check the number, regularity, and strength of the beats. If you notice anything out of the ordinary, make a written note and tell the doctor or home care nurse.

ᴪ If you have been instructed by the doctor to take the pulse, find out what pulse range is normal and what rate you should report to the doctor. Keep a written record of the pulse rates and take it with you to the next doctor's appointment.

Respiration

Respiration is the act or process of breathing.

ᴪ Sometimes the person will have a tendency to breathe more deliberately when he knows you are counting his respirations. You can alleviate this problem by counting respirations immediately after taking the pulse. Leave your fingers in position on the wrist and begin to count respirations. He won't be aware that you are counting respirations.

ᴪ Watch the rise and fall of the chest and count the number of respirations during a full one minute period. Breathing in and breathing out counts as one respiration. The normal rate for adults is 16-20 breaths per minute.

ᴪ Check the regularity, depth, effort, and sound of the person's breathing. Report any changes or unusual characteristics to the doctor or home care nurse.

How to Take A Blood Pressure Reading

Blood pressure measures the force that blood exerts against the walls of the blood vessels. Factors that can influence blood pressure readings include medications, exercise, emotions, pain, and stress.

- Several devices are available for taking blood pressure readings in the home. The instruments described here are the traditional sphygmomanometer and stethoscope.

- The sphygmomanometer has a cuff, rubber bulb, and a dial (aneroid) gauge or a vertical mercury gauge.

- The stethoscope is a listening device that magnifies sound.

- Blood pressure is taken by recording two readings. The first reading is called systolic pressure, the pressure felt in the artery when the heart contracts, pumping blood. The second reading is diastolic pressure, the pressure felt in the artery when the heart is in the relaxed stage, filling with blood. The systolic number is always higher than the diastolic number.

- An average normal blood pressure reading is 120/80, but readings vary depending on age, sex, emotional state, fitness, and weight.

- Before taking the person's blood pressure, wash your hands.

- Ask the person to sit or lie in a comfortable position.

ꙮ Place one arm of the person in a resting position at the level of the heart, with the palm of the hand up.

ꙮ If the person has had a stroke, mastectomy, is receiving IV fluids, or is having home dialysis, use the unaffected or uninjured arm only.

ꙮ Remove clothing from the arm.

ꙮ Put the stethoscope around your neck.

ꙮ Sometimes there is air remaining in the cuff of the sphygmomanometer. The cuff should not have air in it. To release the air, open the valve at the bulb by turning it counterclockwise. Squeeze the blood pressure cuff to expel any air. Then close the valve on the bulb by turning it clockwise.

ꙮ Locate the brachial artery by feeling the pulse on the inner side of the elbow with your fingertips.

ꙮ Wrap the cuff securely around the person's arm, one inch above the elbow, with the arrow on the cuff pointing toward the brachial artery.

ꙮ Fasten the cuff snugly, but not tightly.

ꙮ Place the dial gauge on the top of the cuff, or on a stable surface where it is easy to read.

ꙮ Locate the brachial artery again with your fingertips.

ꙮ Place the round disc of the stethoscope over the brachial artery.

ꙮ Insert the stethoscope ear pieces into your ears.

ꙮ Using the rubber bulb and watching the dial gauge,

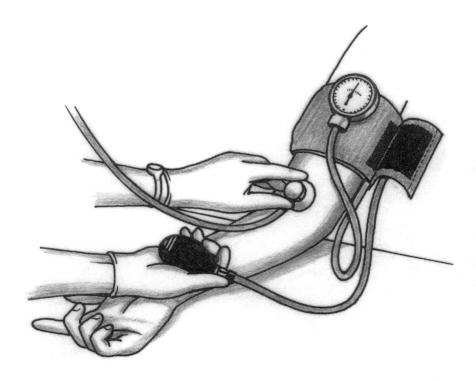

pump air into the cuff until the reading on the gauge is about 200.

- Listen through the stethoscope.
- While listening through the stethoscope, slowly and evenly release the air by turning the valve on the rubber bulb counterclockwise. If air escapes too fast, the reading on the dial or gauge will drop quickly, and you will have to tighten the bulb valve or start over.

🌭 Listen closely, keeping your eyes on the meter. The first sharp thump you hear indicates the systolic pressure. Note the number on the gauge; it will be the top number of the blood pressure reading when you record it later.

🌭 Keep listening through the stethoscope and reading the gauge as the meter continues to fall. The last thumping sound you hear indicates the diastolic pressure. Remember the number; it will be the bottom number in the reading.

🌭 Allow the remaining air to escape from the cuff.

🌭 Remove the cuff, leaving the valve open.

🌭 Record the blood pressure reading.

🌭 Wash your hands.

🌭 If you are unsuccessful in obtaining a reading after your first attempt, try the same procedure on the other arm. If the blood pressure is difficult to take or if you feel unsure about the procedure or results, consult with the doctor or the home care nurse.

Measuring and Recording Fluid Intake and Output

🌭 The doctor or nurse may ask you to measure the amount of fluid a person takes in and the amount of fluid he or she voids.

🌭 Ice, water, juices, pop, coffee, tea, milk, ice cream, yogurt, soup, jello, pudding, and any other food that is liquid at room temperature is measured.

🖉 Use a note pad to record the time, type of fluid, and the amount of fluid a person drinks. These are intake measurements.

🖉 Output measurements may include urine, liquid stools, vomit, and blood or drainage from wounds.

🖉 Ask the person to use a urinal or bedpan at all times, so you can record the amounts. If he or she can use a toilet, a special plastic insert can be placed in the toilet to collect urine or stools.

🖉 Wash your hands and put on disposable gloves when you measure output.

🖉 Measure and record each kind of output separately.

🖉 Use a large measuring cup or special measuring container to measure output fluids. Pour from the bedpan, urinal, or toilet insert into the cup or container and record the output. Empty fluids into the toilet and flush.

🖉 Clean equipment after each use.

Oxygen Safety

Oxygen equipment is the most hazardous home medical equipment. The pure oxygen in an oxygen cylinder can feed a fire's growth very quickly.

🖉 When oxygen is in use, NO SMOKING and OXYGEN IN USE signs should be posted in plain view at each entryway to the home and at the door of the person's room. The no smoking rule must be strictly enforced.

🌿 Move oxygen cylinders carefully. The cylinders should lie flat or stand secured to a fixed object.

🌿 Keep oxygen cylinders away from combustible materials of any kind. Store them away from the sun and other heat sources.

🌿 Avoid using electrical appliances where oxygen is in use. Any appliance that can produce a spark (such as space heaters, electric razors, and hair dryers) can cause oxygen to ignite.

🌿 Do not use matches, lighters, candles, or open flames where oxygen is in use.

🌿 Avoid using woolen blankets, which may cause sparks from static electricity.

🌿 Do not handle oxygen cylinders with oily hands or gloves because of fire danger.

How to Care for Someone on Oxygen Therapy

🌿 Oxygen is delivered through a tube that runs from the oxygen source to a face mask or nasal cannula.

🌿 The prongs on the nasal cannula should be in the person's nose. Some people experience irritation around the nostrils and the top of the ears when using a nasal cannula. Inspect these areas regularly and report any skin irritation or breakdown to the nurse. Check to be sure that the straps on the cannula are secure, but not too tight. Non-petroleum ointment and padding at the ears can help with irritation.

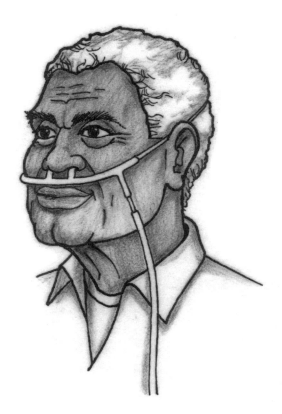

🍂 When checking the face mask, make sure that it covers the nose and mouth and that the interior surface is dry. If the mask is damp or wet, dry it with a clean paper towel before replacing it. Check the skin where the mask touches the face for any irritation. Inform the nurse of any irritation or broken skin.

🍂 Check that the oxygen is being delivered at the correct rate. Adjust the gauge if necessary.

🍂 Elevate the person's head to make breathing easier.

🍂 Oxygen is a dry gas, and it usually passes through a

humidifier that is attached to the oxygen equipment. This adds moisture to the oxygen. Humidifiers must be cleaned and refilled regularly. Follow all the directions given to you by the manufacturer or by the doctor or nurse.

✷ Oxygen may dry the membranes of the mouth and respiratory system, even with a humidifier. Provide frequent mouth care, apply a non-petroleum lubricant to the lips if necessary, and encourage the person to drink plenty of fluids.

When to Call 911

Sometimes it's hard to know when to call for help. Here is a list of conditions that require emergency services:

- Severe bleeding
- Seizure
- Paralysis
- Vomiting blood or bleeding from the rectum
- Possible broken bones after a fall
- Slurred speech
- Persistent pressure or severe pain in the abdomen
- Difficulty breathing
- No pulse and no breathing
- Chest pain or pressure in the chest
- Particular danger signs associated with a heart attack include: radiating pain from the chest down into the arms, up the neck to the jaw, and into the back; crushing, squeezing chest pain or heavy pressure in the chest, shortness of breath, excessive sweating, bluish and pale skin, nausea, vomiting, and weakness.

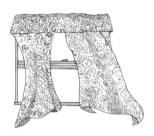

Chapter 7
How to Manage Medications

Drugs and the Elderly

Older people have an average of four chronic diseases (such as arthritis, high blood pressure, heart disease, and diabetes) being treated at any one time. Each disease may require multiple medications to relieve the symptoms.

- 🕯 People 65 years or older take an average of 8 drugs per day. The more medications taken, the greater the risk of medication errors and drug interactions.

- 🕯 Aging changes the way our bodies absorb, metabolize, respond to, and eliminate medications.

- 🕯 Decreased gastric acids in the stomach reduce absorption of some foods or drugs.

- Older adults take longer to absorb oral medications, and it takes longer for the medication to work.

- Our intestines digest more slowly and drug absorption is delayed.

- Certain diseases affect the efficiency and speed of the intestines.

- Laxatives may increase intestinal activity, reducing the absorption of medications.

- The total volume of blood and water in the body decreases as our bodies age. The effects of a medication may be stronger because it is distributed through the body in a more concentrated form.

- Dehydration, a common problem among the elderly, also concentrates medication.

- At age 70, people have 25% more body fat than they do at age 40, even if they maintain the same weight. Fat soluble drugs are more likely to be dissolved and stored in fat reservoirs instead of circulating in the blood, delaying drug action, breakdown, and elimination.

- With age, responses to medication become more varied and unpredictable.

- People who are 60-70 years old are twice as likely to have an undesirable drug reaction as are people who are 30-40 years old.

- In older people, the kidneys and liver break down and eliminate medications from the body more slowly. The drug remains active in the body for a longer time, with potentially negative effects.

🍂 Drugs are tested by and formulated for a younger, healthier age group, but are generally used by the chronically ill older adult.

🍂 It is very important that medications given to the elderly be monitored carefully.

When to Manage Someone's Medications

You should manage medications when:

🍂 The person's physical impairment makes it difficult for him to access the medications.

🍂 He has difficulty opening containers.

🍂 His sense of touch is impaired. He picks up more than one pill at a time without realizing it.

🍂 His vision impairment makes it difficult for him to read a label or understand how to take a medication. He may not be able to distinguish medications by color.

🍂 He is mentally or cognitively challenged. He forgets to take his medicine. He has difficulty understanding why he is taking the medication, or denies the need for it as soon as he feels better.

🍂 He is taking several different kinds of medicine at different times throughout the day. He has difficulty coping with the complicated medication schedule.

🍂 He is taking over-the-counter drugs with prescription medications and the doctor may not be aware of the situation.

🌿 He has difficulty going to the pharmacy to pick up prescription refills.

🌿 He is being treated by more than one physician or using more than one pharmacy.

🌿 He has the most common medication problem seen in the elderly, the underuse of medicine.

🌿 He uses outdated medicine, or fails to refill a prescription.

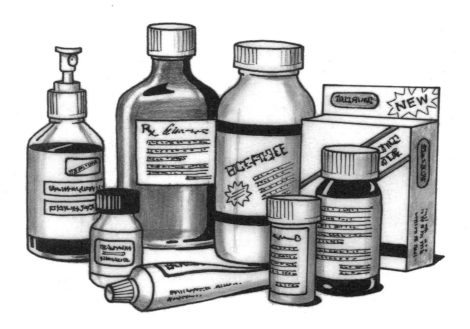

At the Doctor's Office

When you visit the doctor, bring a list of all current medications. The list should include vitamins and nutritional supplements, natural herbal products, ear and eye drops, inhalers, suppositories, ointments, alcohol, caffeine, nicotine, and over-the-counter drugs, as well as all prescription drugs. Some drug combinations should not be taken, and there may be drugs that should be discontinued. Bring a pen and notebook to write down the answers to questions you ask the doctor.

Questions to Ask the Doctor

If the doctor prescribes new medication, here are some important questions to ask:

- Can the medication be prescribed in the less expensive generic form? Find out both the drug's brand name and generic name.

- What is the medication supposed to do? Ask the doctor to write the purpose of the medication on the prescription.

- How is the medication given, and how much of the medication should be given each time?

- When, and for how long, should this medication be taken?

- Is the medication to be taken on a full or on an empty stomach? What foods, if any, need to be avoided? Can I crush the medication for easier swallowing?

- Where and how do I store the medicine?

- What do I do if a dose has been missed because it has been vomited, refused, or forgotten?

- Will this drug replace another drug that is currently being used?

❧ Ask the primary care doctor if he or she will coordinate all the medications. If the person has several doctors, ask each one to check with the primary care doctor before prescribing a new medication. Each doctor needs to be aware of all the medications that are being taken.

At the Pharmacy

Your pharmacist is a resource for information, guidance, and help with scheduling medications.

❧ Use only one pharmacy. This allows the pharmacist to evaluate all the drugs taken, and this knowledge will reduce the chance for adverse reactions from drug interactions.

❧ Ask the pharmacist to write out complicated directions.

❧ Ask the pharmacist to help you with the times the medication is given. If a medication needs to be taken on an empty stomach, the pharmacist can tell you how long to wait before or after a meal.

❧ If the medicine has a different size, color, or shape when you refill a prescription, ask the pharmacist to explain the difference before you give the medicine.

❧ Ask the pharmacist to answer any questions that the doctor did not answer.

❧ Before leaving the pharmacy, look at the package for signs of tampering such as broken seals, open or damaged wrappings, or puncture holes. Check the label to be sure it is the correct drug and that the directions for use are clear.

Side Effects and Adverse Reactions

❧ A side effect is a common, known, expected response to medication. Antihistamines, for example, are known to cause drowsiness.

❧ An adverse reaction is an unwanted, harmful, or unexpected response to a medication.

❧ Most adverse reactions occur as a result of interaction with food or other drugs, or as a result of an allergic reaction to a drug or combination of drugs.

❧ Over-the-counter drugs, alcohol, caffeine, and natural herbal products are drugs that can cause adverse reactions when combined or used with prescription medications. Check with the doctor before giving any over-the-counter drugs.

❧ Symptoms of an adverse reaction are not always immediate. They may develop over a period of weeks or months. If an adverse reaction should occur, write down a detailed description and make an accurate report to the doctor or nurse as soon as possible. Some typical signs of an adverse reaction to medication include:

- Tremors or stiffness
- Indigestion, constipation, diarrhea, or vomiting
- Loss of bladder control or difficulty urinating
- Blurred or double vision

- Loss of hearing or exaggerated hearing
- Dry mouth
- Fatigue or weakness
- Poor appetite
- Difficulty concentrating, forgetfulness, confusion, or depression

❧ Do not assume that confusion or forgetfulness in an elderly person is a natural part of aging. It may be an adverse reaction to medication. He or she should be evaluated by the doctor.

Safe Medication Practices

❧ Do not give someone medication originally intended for another person.

❧ Do not remove medicine from the prescription bottle into another container or pour medications from one bottle to another.

❧ Never stop giving a medication without telling the doctor. There are several reasons for this. Some medications need to be taken for the full length of time prescribed, even after the symptoms are gone. Other medications need to be tapered off. It can take weeks before the results of some medications begin to appear. When one medication is stopped, other medications a person is taking may need to be adjusted.

❧ Never assume that if one pill works well, two will work better.

❧ Any person taking blood thinners, heart medications, and medications for diabetes or seizures should wear a medical alert identification. These medical alert IDs come in bracelet and necklace form and are available at most drug stores.

❧ Medication containers are available that allow you to set up a day or week's worth of medication at one time. Weekly and daily containers are available at most drug stores.

❧ Arrange the medication schedule to coincide with daily events such as meal times, afternoon nap times, and bedtime. Those are the times when taking medication will be easiest to remember.

❧ Automatic medication dispensing systems that are preprogrammed to dispense medication at regular intervals are also available. A sound similar to that of an alarm clock alerts the person that it is time to take the medication, and the machine automatically dispenses the appropriate medicine. Some of these units can be connected to a monitoring center: if the medication is not taken within 30 minutes, the device will automatically alert the monitoring center and someone will call you or the person directly. These machines are not appropriate for someone with dementia. Another person needs to be responsible for administering medications to someone who has dementia.

❧ If you hire someone privately or ask a friend or another family member to help, you can teach that person how to set up and give the medications.

💌 An agency home health aide is prohibited by law from administering medications of any kind, whether prescription or over-the-counter.

💌 Wash your hands before you begin to prepare medicine.

General Guidelines for Administering Medications

THE FIVE R's

Keep the 5 R's in mind whenever you administer medication. Ask yourself, is this:

1. **The right medication?**
2. **The right person?**
3. **The right time?**
4. **The right dose?**
5. **The right route?**

💌 Avoid distractions. Make sure you have adequate lighting.

💌 Never give medication from an unlabeled container.

💌 Check the expiration date on the prescription label. If the medicine is outdated, do not use it.

💌 Check the label again to see that it contains the name of the person for whom it is intended. Check that it is the correct medication, the proper dosage, and the proper time before you remove the drug from the container.

❦ Look at the medicine itself. If it appears discolored, has an unusual odor, or seems suspicious in any way, do not give it.

❦ Avoid touching medications. Remove a dose of the medicine from its container by dropping it into a spoon or the container's cap. Then drop the medication into a cup or small saucer.

❦ Read the label a third time and check the 5 R's again before you return the container to the shelf.

❦ Use a spoon to place the medication into the person's mouth, or hand her a cup with the medication in it and let her take the medicine on her own.

❦ Watch the person until you are sure she has taken the drug.

❦ Record the date, time, and dosage in a medication log immediately after you have given medicine. Take the medication log with you when you visit the doctor.

Administering Different Forms of Medication

Oral Medication

❦ Always wash your hands before giving medication.

❦ Oral medications, given by mouth, usually come in pill or capsule form.

❦ Water is the safest liquid to use when giving oral

medications. Milk and some juices can interfere with absorption.

🌿 Pills tend to stick in a mouth that is dry. Offer a sip of water before giving the medication.

🌿 Don't chew, crush, or break capsules or tablets unless you have first checked with your pharmacist.

🌿 If you have been instructed to crush the medication, pill crushers are available at most drug stores. Place the crushed medication in 1 tablespoon of applesauce and mix. Make sure that the person swallows all of the applesauce.

🌿 Use a pill cutter or splitter if you have been instructed to give half a tablet.

Liquid Medication

🌿 Always wash your hands before giving medication.

🌿 Many liquid medications need to be shaken. Check the label for instructions.

🌿 To keep the label clean and easy to read, pour liquid medications with the label facing upward.

🌿 Avoid using household spoons. Use measuring spoons instead.

🌿 If a calibrated spoon or cup is provided with the liquid medication, it should be used with that liquid only.

Sublingual Medication

🌿 Always wash your hands before giving medication.

🌿 Sublingual means under the tongue. The medication is absorbed through the lining of the mouth.

🌿 Place the medication under the tongue and let it slowly dissolve.

🌿 Advise the person not to swallow until the tablet has completely dissolved.

Topical Medication

🌿 Always wash your hands before giving medication.

🌿 Topical medications are absorbed through the skin surface.

🌿 Apply the ointment using a cotton-tipped swab, or, while wearing gloves, apply the ointment with your fingertips. Ointments should not be applied too thickly.

🌿 Consult the doctor if any redness or irritation appears.

Patches

🌿 Patches allow medication to be absorbed slowly through the skin.

🌿 Never cut a patch in half.

🌿 Medication patches should be applied at the same time each day.

🌿 Wash your hands. Try not to touch the medicine on the patch when you apply it.

🌿 Apply the patch to a new area each time. Avoid areas that are hairy or oily. The most common areas for patches are the upper arms, shoulders, chest, abdomen, and back.

✺ Press the patch firmly into place with the palm of your hand.

✺ Wash your hands.

Inhalers

Medication Nebulizer

✺ When discharging medication from the nebulizer into the mouth, the person should breathe normally, taking a deep breath from time to time.

✺ It may take up to 15 minutes for medication to be discharged completely from the bulb of the nebulizer.

Metered-Dose Inhaler

✺ Shake the pressurized canister for 15 seconds to make certain that the medication is ready to be dispensed.

✺ Hold the device about 1 inch away from the mouth.

✺ Exhale.

✺ Activate the device by pressing the top of the pressurized canister.

✺ Inhale as the medication is released, breathing in the medication. Have the person hold his or her breath before exhaling.

✺ If more than one dose is prescribed, wait 30 seconds between doses.

❧ The metered-dose inhaler is difficult for many people to use because of poor hand-eye coordination or difficulty in discharging the device while inhaling.

❧ A holding chamber or spacer can be attached to the inhaler to prevent problems in administering the medication.

❧ With the holding chamber attached, the person simply discharges the medication into the holding chamber and breathes the medication in slowly.

Eye Drops

❧ Wash your hands before administering medication and wear disposable gloves.

❧ Tilt the person's head back slightly. Ask him or her to look up at the ceiling.

❧ Gently pull the lower lid of the eye down. Deposit one drop into the area between the lower lid and the eye.

❧ Place your thumb and forefinger over the inner corner of each eye to prevent the drop from draining into the nasal canal.

❧ If two drops are prescribed for each eye, wait 1-2 minutes before administering the second drop, or it will simply wash out the first drop.

Eye Ointment

❧ Wash your hands before administering medication and wear disposable gloves.

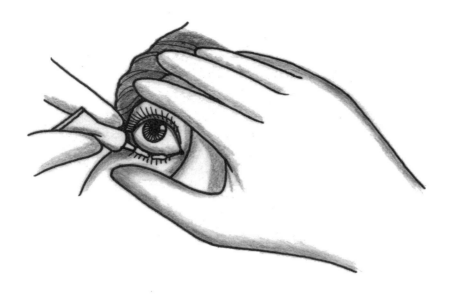

❧ Tilt the person's head back slightly. Ask him or her to look up at the ceiling.

❧ Holding the person's lower lid down, start near the nose and begin to squeeze a line of ointment in the area between the lower lid and the eye. Continue around the outside edge of the lid.

❧ Allow the person to close his or her eye to distribute the medication.

Ear Drops

❧ Wash your hands before administering medications.

❧ Warm the ear drop solution in warm water for 10-15 minutes.

❧ Do not use a microwave oven to heat the ear medication. It could burn the ear.

🌿 Check the instructions to see if the solution needs to be shaken before administering.

🌿 Place the prescribed number of drops in the ear with the head tilted to the side so that the drops can fully enter the ear. With the head still tilted, hold a tissue over the area for one minute.

🌿 Wait a few minutes to allow the medication to be well absorbed in the ear.

Vaginal Suppositories

Suppositories are usually wrapped in foil and kept in the refrigerator. Once the suppository has been inserted, body warmth will melt it in 15- 30 minutes.

🌿 Gather the supplies: disposable gloves, suppository and applicator, water-soluble lubricant, and a protective pad or paper towels.

🌿 Wash your hands and put on the gloves.

🌿 Tell her what you plan to do.

🌿 Ask her to urinate before proceeding.

🌿 Place a towel under the buttocks. She should be lying on her back with knees bent.

🌿 Open the package containing the suppository and place the suppository into the applicator. Lubricate the applicator tip with water-soluble jelly.

🌿 Insert the suppository into the vagina using the applicator plunger.

🌿 Remove the gloves and wash your hands.

Storing Medications

🌿 Keep medication containers tightly closed. Store medications in a cool, dry place, unless instructed otherwise.

🌿 Always read and follow the storage directions printed on the container. Some medications need to be refrigerated.

🌿 Avoid storing medications on windowsills, in the bathroom, or near sinks. Light, heat, and moisture can spoil or decompose some medications.

🌿 Keep creams and skin ointments separate from toothpaste or pills.

🌿 Medications for the eyes, ears, and nose should be stored separately from each other.

🌿 Medicines for pets should be stored separately from medications intended for humans.

🌿 Keep medicines out of the reach of children.

🌿 Do not throw outdated or spoiled medication into household trash accessible to children or pets. Dispose of pills, liquids, and used patches by throwing them into the toilet and flushing immediately.

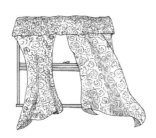

Chapter 8
Nutrition

Nutrition and the Elderly

- One-third of people over 65 suffer from nutritional deficiencies.

- The incidence of protein-calorie malnutrition is higher among the elderly.

- Older adults absorb fewer nutrients from the foods they eat and the ability to digest fats decreases with age.

- Fewer calories are needed to maintain body weight.

- Anorexia, depression, social isolation, and failure to thrive are common among the elderly; these directly affect eating and nutrition.

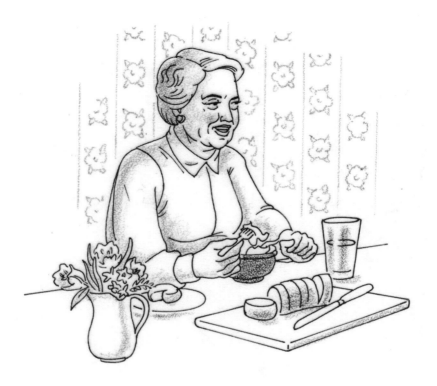

🌿 Loss of appetite because of a decreased ability to taste or smell food is common among the elderly. The inability to smell or taste food can be a result of normal aging or can result from medications and disease.

🌿 Ill-fitting or painful dentures can make eating difficult.

🌿 Some medications can affect how the body absorbs nutrients. For example, habitual use of laxatives can decrease absorption of minerals such as calcium and potassium. Chronic aspirin use has been associated with Vitamin B deficiency.

🦚 People with Alzheimer's or dementia may forget to eat or may lose interest in food, and a lack of transportation may make it difficult for them to shop for food.

🦚 A noisy or chaotic dining environment and frequent interruptions during mealtimes may make eating an unenjoyable event.

Dietary Recommendations for the Elderly

Nutritional needs change at various stages of life. The diet recommendations for the elderly take into account:

🦚 A decreased ability to absorb nutrients and fats.

🦚 Decreased energy needs, which means fewer calories.

🦚 An increased need for nutrient-rich foods.

🦚 An increased need for fiber.

Specialized recommendations for seniors 70 years of age and over according to the USDA Human Nutrition Research Center on Aging, Tufts University, Boston, are:

🦚 Choose the lowest number of recommended servings from each food group.

🦚 For grain products, choose whole grain, enriched/fortified products: brown rice rather than white, and high fiber breakfast cereal fortified with Vitamin B-12 and folic acid.

🦚 Choose whole food rather than juice, and choose fruits and vegetables that are deeply colored: dark green, orange, red and yellow ones should be chosen often.

🌿 Dairy choices should be low in fat, with at least three calcium-rich servings daily or the equivalent in calcium-fortified orange juice or nutritional supplements.

🌿 Choose a variety of lean cuts of meat and poultry from the protein group. Eat fish at least once a week and a legume (dry bean) dish at least twice a week instead of a meat main dish.

🌿 Most fat choices should be limited. Those chosen should consist of a variety of unsaturated liquid oils, rather than hydrogenated or saturated fats.

A Daily Food Guide

The best diet is one high in grain products, fruits and vegetables, and low in saturated fats and cholesterol. Limit foods that contain no nutrient value such as refined sugar, caffeine, and alcohol. According to the United States Department of Agriculture, the recommended food groups are:

Dairy Products (milk, yogurt, cheese) 2-3 serings per day

Protein Foods (meat, dry beans, nuts, eggs) 2-3 servings per day

Fruit or Fruit Juices 2-4 servings per day

Vegetables 3-5 servings per day

Starches (bread, pasta, cereal) 6-11 servings per day

Recommended Serving Sizes

Dairy Products

1 cup of milk or yogurt

1 1/2 ounces natural cheese or 2 ounces of processed cheese

1 1/3 cups of cottage cheese

Protein Foods

2-3 ounces of cooked lean meat, poultry, or fish

1/2 cup of cooked dry beans

1 egg

2 tablespoons peanut butter

1/3 cup nuts

Fruit or Fruit Juices

1 medium apple, banana, orange

1/2 cup of chopped, cooked, or canned fruit

3/4 cup of fruit juice

1/4 cup dried fruit (raisins, prunes, figs)

Vegetables

1 cup of raw leafy vegetables

1/2 cup of other vegetables, cooked or chopped raw

3/4 cup vegetable juice

1 small potato

Starches

 1 slice of bread, 1 ounce of ready-to-eat dry cereal

 1/2 cup of cooked cereal, rice, or pasta

 3-4 crackers

To Decrease Fat in the Diet:

 🌿 Use low-fat or non-fat milk for drinking and cooking.

 🌿 Bake food instead of frying.

 🌿 Trim fat from meat before cooking.

 🌿 Add less fat or oil to food.

 🌿 Eat more fresh fruits and vegetables.

To Decrease Salt in the Diet:

 🌿 Avoid foods high in added salt such as canned vegetables, soups, bouillon cubes, bacon, and cheeses.

 🌿 Use lemon juice, vinegar, garlic, onions, or herbs such as basil, oregano, garlic, and sage to season foods.

The Importance of Water

 Water is vital to health and well being. It is necessary to drink 6-8 cups of water daily. The body needs water to digest, to flush and eliminate toxins, to maintain body temperature, and to prevent dehydration.

 🌿 Many older people suffer from dehydration. Some medications can contribute to dehydration.

 🌿 The thirst response decreases as we age. Older people don't feel thirsty as often.

🌿 People who suffer from incontinence may limit their fluid intake in order to avoid embarrassment.

🌿 Encourage the person in your care to drink fluids, especially water. Serve foods that are high in liquid content, such as watermelon, citrus fruits, tomatoes, cucumbers, and clear soup. Avoid caffeine and alcohol, which can cause dehydration.

Warning Signs of Dehydration

1. The person complains of thirst.
2. The mouth, tongue, lips, and skin will appear dry. The lips may be cracked. The eyes may look sunken.
3. Urinary output is decreased. The urine may be dark amber in color, rather than light yellow. The average urine output is 1 1/2 - 2 quarts per day.
4. Vomiting and diarrhea.
5. Fever and excessive perspiration.

Feeding Someone Who Cannot Feed Himself

🌿 Encourage the person to participate as much as possible.

🌿 Wash your hands. Tell the person what you plan to do.

🌿 Wash his face and hands. Suggest any mouth care that would make eating more desirable. Check to see that dentures, if any, are in place. Bring the person into a sitting position in the bed or preferably in a chair. Drape a napkin over the chest and under the chin. Keep a moistened hand towel nearby for any cleanup.

🌿 Serve food on a tray. Use thermal bowls and cups to keep food at the proper temperature. Bring the food to the person, telling him what you have prepared. Sit near the person.

🌿 Cut food into bite-sized pieces and pour or prepare liquids as necessary.

🌿 Ask the person which food he or she wants first.

🌿 Let him set the pace. Feed one bite at a time, using a half-filled spoon. Place the tip of the spoon to one side of his mouth. Remove the spoon when he has taken the food from the spoon.

🌿 If possible, have the person hold finger foods or bread.

🌿 Use a straw for drinking cool beverages. Wait until he finishes chewing before offering something to drink. Guide the straw or the edge of the cup to his lips.

🌿 Offer praise and encouragement. Mealtime is an excellent time to have conversation.

🌿 When he has finished, wash his hands and face and remove the tray. This is a good time for routine oral hygiene. Clean up any spilled food or drink.

🌿 Keep the person sitting upright for at least 30 minutes after the meal to aid in digestion.

🌿 Wash dishes, utensils, and your own hands.

❧ Decreased appetite and any swallowing difficulties should be reported to the doctor or nurse.

Eating Aids That Can Make Mealtime Easier

❧ Swivel spoons for those with limited wrist movement.

❧ Foam cylinders that fit over and enlarge gripping surfaces of utensils.

❧ Plate guards and high-sided dishes that keep food on the plate and make it easier to scoop food onto utensils.

❧ Rocker knives that cut food using a rocking motion. Small pizza cutters or rolling knives work well.

❧ Food warming dishes for a person who eats slowly.

❧ Rubber-tipped baby spoons and a child's feeder cup or plastic glass.

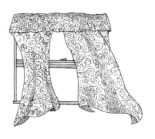

Chapter 9

How to Help Someone Who Uses a Wheelchair

Wheelchair Transfers

Moving someone from one surface area to another is called a transfer. One example of a transfer is moving someone from the bed to a wheelchair. The method used to transfer someone will vary depending on the weight and height of the person being transferred and the person helping to transfer. The amount of assistance varies, too. One person may need only minimal assistance to get in and out of a wheelchair, while another person may need maximum assistance. No one method is right for everyone. If you need to help someone to transfer in and out of a wheelchair, always get instruction from a physical therapist. Ask your doctor for a referral.

- ❧ Flat shoes with a non-skid sole should be worn by you and by the person being transferred.

- ❧ Good lighting is important. Never try to move someone in the dark.

- ❧ Some pets can get underfoot. Place pets in another room before attempting a transfer.

- ❧ Allow the person to help as much as possible.

- ❧ Before attempting a transfer, always tell the person what you are planning to do.

Setting Up the Wheelchair

- ❧ At least half the work of every wheelchair transfer is in the set up: the correct positioning of the wheelchair and the correct positioning of the person you are helping to move.

- ❧ Always begin with the wheelchair on the person's strong side, if there is one.

- ❧ The wheelchair should be set at a 45 degree angle to the bed or whatever surface you are transferring from.

- ❧ Lock both sides of the wheelchair.

- ❧ Swing both foot plates up and away to the raised position or remove them.

How to Transfer Someone from a Bed to a Wheelchair Using a Stand Pivot Transfer

This method of transfer is best used for someone who needs minimal assistance to stand.

- Tell him what you are about to do.
- Follow the instructions for setting up the wheelchair (refer to page 154).
- Help him if necessary to sit at the edge of the bed (refer to page 60).

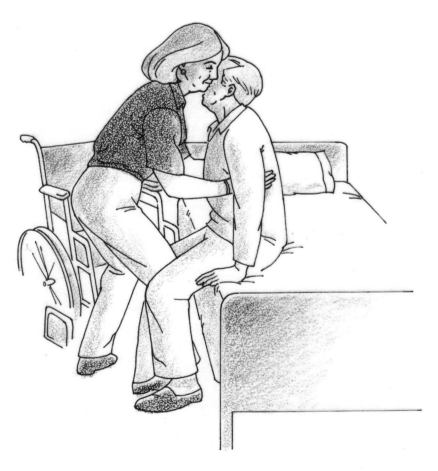

- At the beginning of the transfer, he should be in a sitting position at the edge of the bed with his hips closest to the wheelchair and his knees and feet angled away from the wheelchair.

- Position your foot between his feet and your knee between his knees. Your other foot should be behind about 2 feet back, at a 45 degree angle. Your feet should be about a foot apart.

- Support him by placing your hands underneath and just past his armpits. Position your hands on the sides of his back, fingers pointing toward each other.

- Ask him to place his hands on the bed to help push up (See illustration page 155).

- Count 1-2-3 together out loud and on the count of 3, have him lean over slightly as he shifts his weight forward from his buttocks to his feet and pushes up with his hands. Shift your weight onto your back leg at the same time. Keep your back straight and knees bent. Help him into a standing position with one smooth continuous motion.

- When standing, support his lower back with your hands. Give him a moment to adjust in case of dizziness or imbalance.

- Continue to support him as he takes small steps, slowly turning toward the wheelchair.

- Stop when he can feel the edge of the chair seat on the back of both of his legs.

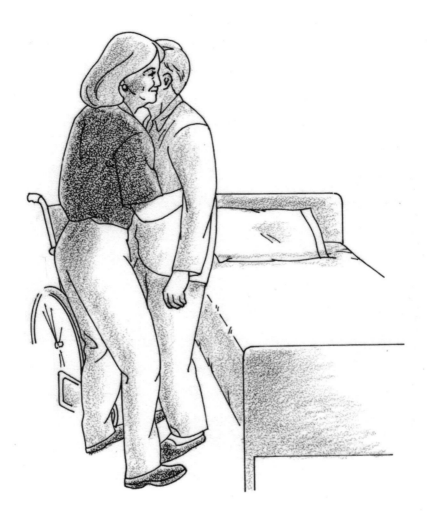

🍃 With his knees slightly bent, have him reach back and put one hand on each armrest of the chair to guide himself into the chair.

🌿 Keep your back straight, bend your knees, and use your leg muscles as you help to lower him into the chair.

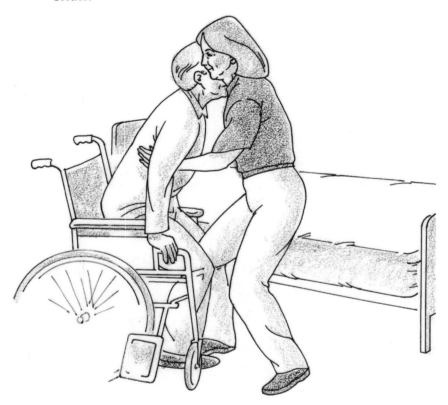

Gait Belt

A gait belt is a sturdy cloth strap, measuring about three inches wide and three feet long. Also known as a walking belt or transfer belt, it is a supportive aid used to help a weak or unsteady person to transfer or walk. You can hold onto the gait belt to give support when transferring a person from one position to another.

Applying and Using a Gait Belt in a Stand Pivot Transfer (Bed to Wheelchair)

The gait belt gives you more control of the person's body. It is helpful when assisting someone who has difficulty moving into a standing position.

- ❦ Tell the person what you are about to do.

- ❦ Follow the instructions for setting up the wheelchair (refer to page 154).

- ❦ Assist the person to a sitting position at the side of the bed (refer to page 60).

- ❦ Place the gait belt around the hips over clothing. Some people find it easier to position the gait belt over the waist. Never place a gait belt over bare skin, drains, feeding tubes, or a colostomy.

- ❦ Tighten the belt until it is snug but comfortable. It should not create breathing difficulties or discomfort.

- ❦ At the beginning of the transfer, he should be in a sitting position at the edge of the bed with his hips closest to the wheelchair and his knees and feet angled away from the wheelchair.

- ❦ Position your foot between his feet and your knee between his knees. Your other foot should be behind about 2 feet back at a 45 degree angle. Your feet should be about a foot apart.

- ❦ Ask him to place his hands on the bed to help push up.

- ❦ Hold onto the gait belt at his waist with both hands.

✹ Count 1-2-3 together and on the count of 3, have him lean over slightly as he shifts his weight forward from his buttocks to his feet and pushes up with his hands. Shift your weight onto your back leg at the same time. Keep your back straight and knees bent. Help him into a standing position with one continuous movement.

✹ Continue to support him by holding the gait belt as he steps toward the wheelchair.

✹ Stop when he can feel the edge of the chair seat on the back of both of his legs.

✹ With his knees slightly bent, have him reach back and put one hand on each armrest of the chair to guide himself into the chair.

✹ Keep your back straight, bend your knees, and use your leg muscles as you help to lower him into the chair.

Transferring a Person into a Vehicle

✹ Open the car door as far as possible and move the front seat of the car as far back as possible.

✹ Swing the foot supports out of the way or remove them. If you remove the foot support closest to the car, you will be able to move the chair as close to the car as possible.

✹ Place the wheelchair at a 45 degree angle to the car seat and set both of the wheel locks. The person should be sitting at the edge of the wheelchair.

🌿 Position your knee that is farthest from the car door between his knees, with your other leg back at a 45 degree angle. If there isn't enough room, bend your knees and position your feet in a wide stance, keeping your center of gravity as low as you can to protect your back.

🌿 Support him by placing your hands underneath and just past his armpits. Position your hands on the sides of his back, fingers pointing toward each other. If you are using a gait belt, grasp the belt at both sides of his waist.

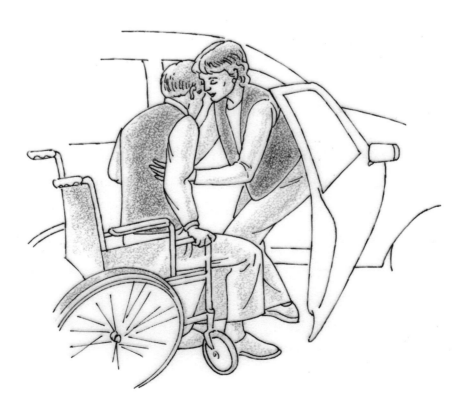

❧ Have him place his hands on the armrests of the wheelchair to help push up.

❧ Count 1-2-3 together and on the count of 3, help him to stand as he shifts his weight from his buttocks to his feet and pushes up with his hands. Use your legs, not your back, to help him into a standing position in one smooth continuous motion.

❧ Give him a few moments to adjust to the standing position.

❧ Support him while he takes small steps, turning toward the seat of the car.

❧ Protect his head and neck with one arm as you lower him into the car seat. Be aware of your body position. Bend at your knees; let your legs do the work, not your back.

❧ If necessary, help him lift his legs into the car.

Loading the Wheelchair into the Car

❧ Remove the foot plates and armrests and load them into the car first. This will eliminate some of the weight of the wheelchair.

❧ Fold the wheelchair and lock it in the collapsed position.

❧ Keep the chair as close to your body as possible.

❧ Use your legs to lift the chair into the car, while keeping your back straight.

How to Maneuver Ramps and Curbs

❧ When going down a ramp, go backwards, keeping your body between the wheelchair and the low end of the ramp. Keep your legs bent as you maneuver the chair down the ramp.

❧ When negotiating curbs, move the front of the wheelchair as close to the curb as possible. Use the tip bars located at the back and bottom part of the wheelchair to tip the front wheels onto the curb. Lift the rear wheels up the curb as you move the wheelchair forward. Use your legs to do the lifting.

❧ When going down a curb, go backwards. Position yourself with your back and the back of the wheelchair at the edge of the curb. Step down and lower the rear wheels first, and then use the tip bars to gently lower the front wheels.

Helping Someone to Walk with or without a Gait Belt

Walking is highly beneficial for maintaining health, independence, and a positive mood. If a person's condition allows, walk with him or her several times a day, even if it is only for short distances.

❧ Clear obstacles from the pathway before you begin.

❧ If you are using a gait belt, position it around the person's hips over the clothing. Some people find it easier to place the gait belt around the waist. Never use a gait belt over bare skin, drains, feeding tubes, or a colostomy.

- Tighten the belt until it is snug but comfortable. It should not create breathing difficulties or discomfort.

- Stand slightly behind and to one side of the person, holding onto the gait belt at each side of his waist. If you are walking without a gait belt, support him with one hand around his waist and the other supporting his elbow and forearm.

- Taking small steps, assist the person to walk.

- Encourage him to go a few more steps than he did during the previous walk.

How to Assist a Person Who Is Falling

Whenever you assist someone to walk, there is always a possibility that he or she could become weak, dizzy, or could stumble and fall. Never try to catch the person or stop the fall. It is better to assist the fall by helping him to the floor.

- A good position for assisting someone who is falling is standing slightly behind and to one side of the person, supporting him at the waist.

- As he starts to fall, quickly place your feet at shoulder's width apart to provide a stable base. Keep your knees slightly bent and your back straight.

- Place your arms around the person's waist or under his arms. If the person is wearing a gait belt, grasp the gait belt for support.

- Pulling his body toward you, position one of your

legs forward with your knee bent to serve as a rest for the person's buttocks.

🌿 Let his buttocks rest on your knee.

🌿 Allow him to slide slowly down your leg, as you bend at the knees and hips.

🌿 Protect the head of the person as he comes to rest on the floor.

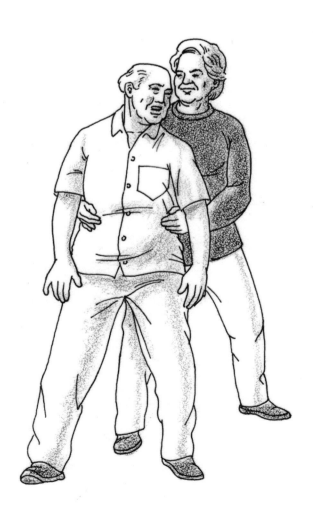

❧ If the fall occurred from dizziness or light-headedness, allow him to relax for a few moments.

❧ Help the person to crawl to the nearest piece of stable furniture. He can use the furniture to help himself to get up. Assist him if necessary.

❧ If the person becomes unconscious, call 911.

Reporting a Fall

❧ Falling can be a sign of a serious medical condition such as pneumonia, urinary tract infection, or heart problems. It is important to report all falls to the doctor.

❧ Record the day, time, location of the fall, how the fall occurred, and any history of previous falls. This information can help the doctor to determine if the fall was a result of medications, Sundowner's Syndrome, vision problems, an activity, or hazards in the home.

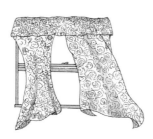

Chapter 10
Fall Prevention

Each year, 1 out of every 3 people over the age of 65 has a fall. Falls are the leading cause of death from injury for people 65 years or older. The most common form of injury from a fall is a hip fracture.

🌿 The emotional effects of a fall can be devastating. Fear of falling again can cause a person to restrict his or her activities, resulting in feelings of loss, loneliness, and helplessness. Avoiding activity because of fear and anxiety can actually increase the risk of falling again.

🌿 Try not to contribute to the fear of falling by putting too many restrictions on activities.

❧ Encourage regular exercise and enjoyable activities that promote independence. A primary goal of fall prevention is maintaining and encouraging independence.

❧ Medical conditions that contribute to falls should be treated by the doctor. Vision and hearing should be checked regularly.

❧ Remove hazards in and around the home. Alert visitors to hazards that cannot be removed, such as oxygen tubing.

❧ Don't assume that falls and the problems that lead to falls are a natural, unavoidable part of the aging process.

Protecting Yourself from Falls

❧ Never carry objects that are too heavy or large, making balance difficult.

❧ When carrying objects, do not allow your vision to be blocked. Make more trips with smaller loads.

❧ Take the time to position your body correctly, using proper body mechanics whenever you move objects or help someone to move.

❧ Never rush to do your tasks or hurry the person for whom you are caring.

Proper Shoes

❧ Shoes should have low heels and a good tread.

❧ Avoid smooth leather soles or tennis shoes with a smooth bottom.

꙰ Periodically check the soles of your shoes and those of the person in your care to see if they have worn smooth.

꙰ Keep shoelaces tied or Velcro firmly fastened.

꙰ Shoes with high tops will help prevent a twisted ankle, especially when walking on uneven surfaces.

꙰ Shoe chains or studded traction soles help to prevent slipping on ice or snow.

꙰ Slippers should have rubber soles. Do not wear slippers outside.

꙰ Stocking feet are very slippery and should be avoided.

Fall-Proofing the Home

꙰ Area rugs and runners should have rubberized non-slip backing.

꙰ Patterned rugs can affect depth perception, especially for the elderly. Solid colored rugs are less confusing.

꙰ Electric cords that run through walkways may cause someone to trip. Place electric cords along the wall.

꙰ Do not place cords or wires under rugs or runners. Uneven surfaces can cause tripping.

꙰ Keep floors clear of clutter. Magazines are slippery. Toys for children or pets can be hazardous.

꙰ Furniture and objects that blend into the carpet, such as glass-topped coffee tables, can be a hazard.

꙰ Use non-slip rubber adhesive under furniture legs to prevent sliding.

- Highly polished waxed floors are very slippery and shiny. Use products that are non-skid and non-glare.

- Clean up spills immediately after they occur.

- Shelves that are too high can result in a fall from bending, overreaching, standing on tiptoes, or using a chair or ladder. Place items that are used regularly between hip and eye level.

- Use a reacher (available at home medical supply stores) for items which are out of comfortable reach.

Bedroom Safety

- The bed should be a comfortable height, stable, and firm enough to get in and out of easily.

- Place a telephone and lamp on the bedside table, within reach of the person in bed. Keep a flashlight on the bedside table for emergencies.

- Eyeglasses, canes, and walkers should be kept within reach.

- Keep electric blanket and heating pad cords out of the way so they don't become a tripping hazard.

- Avoid dresses, pants, and robes that are too long and loose. They can cause someone to trip.

- Have the person sit when dressing or undressing if he or she is unstable when standing.

- High or low blood pressure can cause dizziness, especially when a person gets up from a bed or chair. If dizziness occurs, encourage the person to sit for a few minutes before moving to the standing position.

Bathroom Safety

- Bathrooms are a common area for falls because of water, soapy tile, or porcelain surfaces. Rubberized slip-resistant mats both inside and outside of the shower or tub help prevent slipping.

- Sinks, toilets, and towel bars should be securely fastened.

- Place slip-resistant grab bars inside and outside the shower and tub area and next to the toilet. Grab bars need to be installed correctly. Your home supply store, home care nurse, or therapist can advise you on proper placement and installation.

- Use a shower bench or chair for someone who is unsteady on his or her feet. This will allow the person to sit while showering. The chair or bench should have a back support and rubber-tipped feet to keep it from sliding.

- A raised toilet seat will make it easier and safer for someone who is weak or has balance problems. Some come with armrests.

Proper Lighting

- An older adult needs 3 times more light to see clearly than someone younger. Proper lighting helps to prevent falls.

- Light switches should be accessible at room entrances and at the beginning of any dark area.

- Low wattage bulbs make it hard to see. Always use

the maximum wattage suggested by the manufacturer of the light fixture.

🌿 Auto touch lights that turn on when you touch the base of the lamp are helpful for those with arthritis or painful joints. Adapters are available that will turn your existing lamp into a touch-sensitive lamp.

Stair Safety

🌿 Stairs are the most common place for falls that result in serious injury. Stairs should be well lit so that each step is clearly seen both going up and down, especially the first and last step, the places where most falls occur.

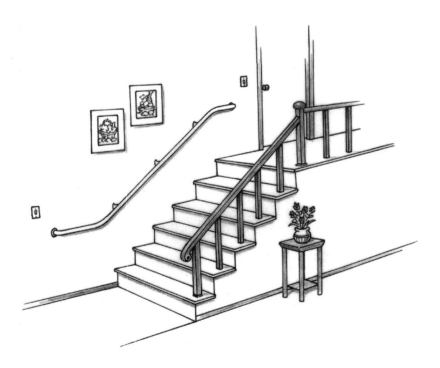

❧ Check carpeted stairs regularly to make sure that the carpet is securely fastened. Check for wrinkles, loose areas, and worn or torn spots that could cause someone to trip.

❧ Do not place loose rugs or runners on the top or bottom of stair landings.

❧ Loose and unstable steps should be repaired or replaced immediately.

❧ All stairways, including outside stairs, should have handrails installed at the correct height on both sides of the stairs. Round handrails are most effective.

Outdoors

❧ Most falls that occur outdoors are on curbs or steps. Step edges should be marked with reflective tape that is designed for outdoor use.

❧ Traction tape on stair treads will minimize the chance of falls when the stairs are wet.

❧ Uneven door thresholds can increase the risk of a fall. Use a contrasting color adhesive strip along the edge of the threshold to make it more visible.

❧ Keep pathways and stairs clean. Leaves, moss, snow, and ice can cause serious falls.

❧ Paths and sidewalks that are raised and cracked create a hazard. Raised areas should be leveled and filled in, and any tree roots removed.

❧ Watch for and replace missing pieces in stone or brick walkways.

❧ Illuminate pathways with exterior lights.

❧ Light larger areas with spotlights.

❧ Keep hoses away from pathways and sidewalks.

❧ Oil or other liquids can make garage floors slippery. Clean all spills immediately. Use a commercial grade oil absorbent for oil spots.

Medications and Fall Risk

Medications can contribute to falls because of side effects such as drowsiness or dizziness. Review medications with the doctor to see if there is increased risk for falls. Some of the drugs that contribute to falls are diuretics, blood pressure medicine, and medications given for psychological reasons.

Sundowner's Syndrome

People with Sundowner's Syndrome behave normally during daylight hours but become confused after the sun goes down. People with Sundowner's are at a greater risk for falls after dark.

Walkers, Canes, and Wheelchairs

Most falls involving walkers and canes result from an improper fit or need for repair. Canes and walkers need to be measured for proper length. Rubber tips should be periodically checked to make sure they are in good condition.

❧ When a person is using a walker, both hands must be free to grasp the handles on either side. Place all packages or small items in a basket or container attached to the walker. Avoid carrying heavy objects, which could cause a loss of balance.

❧ Have wheelchairs checked periodically to make sure they are in good working condition. Never carry heavy objects that can overload a wheelchair.

❧ Always raise or remove the foot supports and lock the wheel locks before transferring.

Emergency Alarm Systems

❧ Alarm systems are available for people who are confused or forgetful and at a high risk for falling. A small transmitter is worn around the thigh or clipped to a collar. When the person wearing the transmitter attempts to walk, crawl, or kneel, the alarm will sound to alert you.

❧ Emergency response systems provide emergency help at the press of a button, 24 hours a day. The response button is worn around the neck, on the belt, or on the wrist. These systems help alleviate the fear of being alone during an emergency such as a fall. They are not appropriate for someone with Alzheimer's disease or dementia: he or she may be confused and forget how to use the alarm.

❧ Contact your local senior programs to find out about available alarm and emergency response systems in your area.

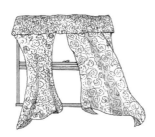

Chapter 11
Fire Safety

Fire safety is an important aspect of home care. More than 400,000 home fires occur in the United States each year, killing more than 4,000 people.

Adults 65 years of age and older are twice as likely to die in a fire than the national average. People 85 years of age and older are 4.5 times more likely to die in a fire.

The Components of a Fire

Four components are necessary for a fire to start:

🔥 The first is oxygen, which is present in the air.

🔥 The second element is fuel: material that will burn, such as cloth, paper, wood, upholstery, or gasoline.

🔥 Heat is the third component. Heat provides the energy necessary for ignition. Common heat sources are stoves, fireplaces, cigarettes, wiring, and furnaces.

🔥 The fourth component is a rapid chemical reaction that occurs when oxygen, fuel, and heat combine.

Reporting a Fire

911 is the number to call for all emergency services in most areas. Check to be sure that your area has 911 service. When reporting a fire:

🔥 Give the dispatcher your name.

🔥 Give your location, including building number, floor, apartment number, and nearest cross street.

🔥 Give the exact location of the fire.

🔥 Give or confirm the phone number you are calling from.

🔥 Remain calm, speak slowly and clearly, and follow any instructions the 911 operator may give you during the call. Stay on the line until the dispatcher tells you to hang up.

Smoke Alarms

According to the United States Fire Administration, 75% of older Americans who die in home fires do not have working smoke alarms. Smoke alarms provide an early warning in the event of a fire, increasing your chance of surviving the fire.

🔥 Smoke alarms should be installed on every level or floor of the house and in every room where people sleep.

🍂 Place the smoke detector on the ceiling at least four inches from the nearest wall (the center of the ceiling is the best placement), away from drafts. The next best place is on the wall 6-12 inches below the ceiling. Follow the manufacturer's instructions for installation and maintenance.

🍂 Each smoke alarm should be tested and vacuumed monthly.

🍂 Check batteries and bulbs at least twice a year.

Using a Fire Extinguisher

🍂 At least one fire extinguisher should be on each level of the home, particularly in the kitchen, garage, laundry room, and workshop.

🍂 Call 911 before attempting to extinguish a fire.

🍂 Plan a clear escape route away from the blaze.

🍂 Stand 6-8 feet away from the fire with your back to your planned escape route and follow the four-step **P.A.S.S.** procedure for extinguishing a fire:
  1) **P**ULL the pin. This unlocks the operating lever and allows you to discharge the extinguisher.
  2) **A**IM low. Point the nozzle or hose at the base of the fire.
  3) **S**QUEEZE the lever above the handle. This discharges the extinguishing agent. Releasing the lever will stop the discharge.
  4) **S**WEEP from side to side. Moving carefully toward the fire, keep the extinguisher aimed at the base

of the fire and sweep back and forth until it appears that the flames are out.

🔥 If the fire reignites, repeat the process.

🔥 Most fire extinguishers last from 8-20 seconds. If you can't control a fire within that time, get out of the house.

🔥 A firefighter needs to inspect the fire site, even if you think the fire is out. Fires can reignite, and firefighters are trained to know what to look for.

When a Person Is on Fire

🔥 Use the stop, drop, and roll technique.

- **Stop** the person from running or walking.
- Help the person **drop** to the floor.
- **Roll** him or her back and forth across the floor several times until the fire is out. Wrapping the person in a blanket can help put the fire out.

Exit Plan

🔥 Time is the critical factor when a fire starts. You have only a few minutes to get yourself and the person in your care to safety. Having a prepared, rehearsed exit plan can mean the difference between life and death.

🔥 Make an escape plan on paper for every family member.

🔥 Draw a floor plan of the house, showing at least two ways out of each room.

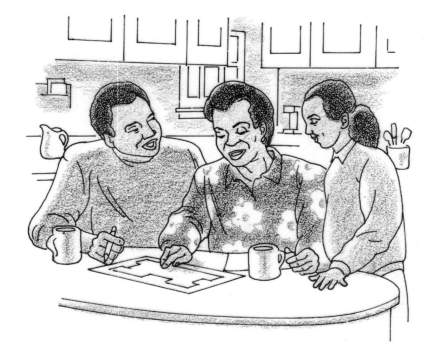

💧 Identify two exits out of the house.

💧 Go over the plan with family members.

💧 Designate a meeting place to gather outside of the home in the event of a fire.

💧 Practice your escape plan at least twice a year. Practice crawling out using the escape plan. Practice in the dark or blindfolded, because fire is black, not light.

💧 Set off the smoke alarm so that everyone knows what it sounds like.

💧 Designate an individual to be responsible for each small child, and for each elderly and disabled person who may not be able to get out of the house on his or her own.

🔥 Become acquainted with your neighbors. They can assist you in getting someone who is disabled out of the house in an emergency.

How to Leave a Burning Building

🔥 Windows and doors to be used as exits should not be obstructed.

🔥 Windows with security bars should be equipped with a quick-release mechanism. Everyone in the house should know how to use the quick-release mechanism.

🔥 Collapsible ladders are available for second floor rooms. The ladder should reach the ground and support the weight of the heaviest person in the home.

🔥 Leave a burning building that is filling with smoke by dropping to your knees and crawling. Less smoke and heat are at floor level. Crawl to the nearest door or window in order to exit the building as quickly as possible.

🔥 Keep your mouth and nose covered with a cloth to avoid breathing smoke and toxic gas.

🔥 Check the safety of a closed interior door during a fire by kneeling or crouching at the door, reaching up as high as you can, and feeling the door with the back of your hand. If it is hot, do not open it. Use another exit route. If the door is cool, brace your shoulder against it and open it carefully and slowly. Close the door behind you. This will help to slow the fire.

🔥 If you are trapped in a burning building, close all the doors between you and the fire and stuff towels, blankets, or rugs in the space between the door and the floor. This will reduce the amount of smoke entering the room.

🔥 If there is a telephone in the room, call 911 and tell the operator your exact location.

🔥 Open a window and breathe the air from the bottom of the window.

🔥 Use the stairway if you are in a burning multi-story building. Never use the elevator: you could become trapped.

🔥 When you are outside, go to the prearranged meeting place.

🔥 If 911 has not yet been called, go to a neighbor's house and call.

Wrap and Slide Technique for Evacuating a Disabled Person

🔥 Use a blanket or sheet to wrap the person's body.

🔥 Grasp the blanket with both hands near the head and shoulders.

🔥 Support the head and shoulders as you gently slide the person off the bed in the direction of the exit.

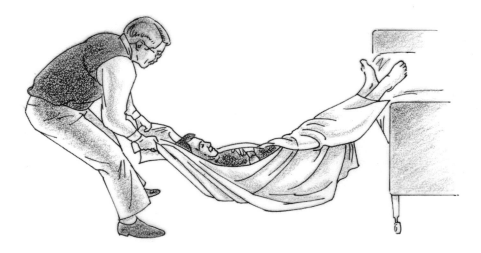

Smoking Safety

🌿 Never leave smoking materials unattended.

🌿 Keep matches and lighters out of direct sunlight and away from heat sources.

🌿 Use wide ashtrays with covers, and keep them away from bedding and other flammable materials.

🌿 Soak the contents of the ashtray and empty them into the toilet before going to bed.

🌿 Carefully check rugs and chair cushions for ashes. Upholstered chairs can smolder for hours before bursting into flame.

🌿 If a cushion or chair has been burned, move it outside away from the house and call the fire department.

❦ Never allow smoking in bed or when lying down.

❦ If the person in your care is confused or has dementia, allow smoking only under supervision.

❦ NEVER allow smoking around oxygen equipment.

❦ Keep smoking materials out of the reach of children.

Home Safety Tips

Kitchen

❦ Keep the stove clean and free of grease build-up.

❦ If a fire starts in a pan, leave the pan on the stove, cover it with a lid and turn off the heat source. Never pour water on a grease fire because it will cause the fire to spread.

❦ Never store anything flammable in the oven or on the range top.

❦ Don't use the stove as an extra heater.

❦ If there is a fire in the oven, keep the oven door closed and call 911.

❦ Avoid using extension cords in the kitchen. Keep electrical cords away from sink areas and hot surfaces.

❦ Avoid wearing loose clothing, especially dangling sleeves that can catch fire while you are cooking. Keep potholders and towels away from the oven and burners.

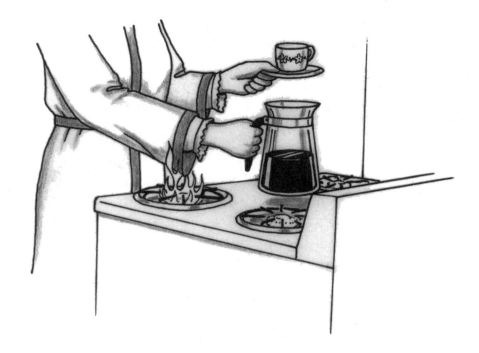

🌿 Prevent burns by turning pot handles inward away from the front of the stove, so they are less likely to be bumped.

🌿 Don't leave cooking unattended, even for short periods of time.

🌿 Avoid placing anything made of metal in the microwave oven. Metal objects will cause sparks that can ignite a fire when the microwave is on.

🌿 Keep a multipurpose, ABC model fire extinguisher in a visible and accessible place.

Bedroom

- ❧ Keep heat sources away from mattresses and bedding.

- ❧ Do not cover or place anything on top of an electric blanket while it is in use.

- ❧ Use heating pads with extreme caution. Heating pads can cause serious burns or fires if left unattended, even on the lowest setting. Never sleep while using a heating pad.

- ❧ Keep a working flashlight, a bell or whistle, eyeglasses, and walking aids within easy reach at the bedside.

- ❧ Close the bedroom door before going to sleep. A closed door helps to slow the spread of a fire.

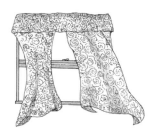

Chapter 12

Elder Neglect and Abuse

One and one-half to two million older adults are esti-mated to be neglected or abused each year. Elderly people with dementia who are living with the caregiver are at a higher risk of abuse than the general population of people over 65.

🍃 Neglect is defined as the failure to provide needed care. When caregivers fail to provide adequate food or clothing, over or under medicate, or leave the older person alone for long periods of time, it is consid-ered neglect.

🍃 Abuse means mistreating or causing harm. It can take physical, emotional, or financial forms. Hitting, slap-ping, kicking, punching, sexual abuse, and confining a person against his or her will are considered physical abuse. Emotional abuse includes using threatening or insulting language which provokes fear, name-calling, treating an elderly person like a child, and intimidating or isolating an elderly person. Financial abuse involves stealing money, checks, and/or possessions, or misusing funds or possessions.

🕊 Abusers are usually family members. Hired caregivers account for 13% of elder abuse.

Causes of elder abuse are often attributed to:

🕊 Alcohol or drug abuse

🕊 Stress from constant caregiving: the psychological and physical demands placed on caregivers. This is especially true of caregivers of those with dementia.

🕊 Refusal of the caregiver to accept or ask for help

🕊 A lack of clear communication

🕊 A family history of violence

🕊 Revenge for earlier abuse done by the older person to the current family caregiver

🕊 Economic factors

🕊 Caregiver perceptions or stereotypes about older people

🕊 Caring for very difficult or abusive people

Family members and victims often try to hide the abuse out of fear or shame. Sometimes it's hard for the abuser to admit his or her own conduct. The behavior is rationalized or downplayed because it is simply too uncomfortable to admit.

Signs of Possible Neglect

- Soiled sheets and clothing that appear to be days old
- Unkept and dirty hair
- Unclean body
- Bedsores
- Trash buildup
- The person complains of no contact with the caregiver
- Filthy bathroom and kitchen areas

Signs of Possible Physical or Sexual Abuse

- Frequent bruises, welts, cuts, sores, or burns to the skin
- Frequent reports of falls
- Broken bones, sprains, dislocations
- Bruises, cuts, or burns in the genital area

Signs of Possible Emotional Abuse

- The care recipient's behavior changes. He or she begins to withdraw, appears depressed, and/or cries frequently.
- The person may appear to be fearful when the caregiver is present or refuse to be left alone with the caregiver.

- The caregiver talks down to, humiliates, or shouts at the person in his or her care.

If you suspect caregiver abuse or neglect, it is your responsibility to report it. Contact the adult protective services of the county department of human services or your state senior and disabled services department. Your suspicions of abuse or neglect will be investigated by a social worker who will make an assessment of the situation.

If you are a caregiver and recognize that you are or have been neglectful or abusive to the person in your care, seek help. The goal of these agencies is to improve the health and safety of the person in your care. The agency is there to provide help to families, not to punish.

Caregiver Abuse

Sometimes it is the caregiver who is being abused by the person he or she is trying to help. Unreasonable demands are made of the caregiver and the person is verbally and/or physically abusive.

- Certain diseases may cause behavior changes that the person is incapable of controlling. His or her attacks or demands are not the person's true nature, but a symptom of the disease. Simply having the understanding that the person has no control over his or her behavior can make it easier to deal with outbursts without taking it personally.

- Caregiver abuse in some situations is intentional. If you are being abused by the person in your care, get help. It is your right to be treated with dignity and respect. The following services can assist you:

- Your primary care doctor
- Home health agency (social worker)
- State senior and disability services
- Area Agency on Aging.
- The community services section in the phone directory.
- The counselor's section in the phone directory. Ask for a referral to a counselor who has experience with caregivers.
- Religious service agencies, clergy or parish nurses.
- Newspaper: Check the events calendar for support group meetings.

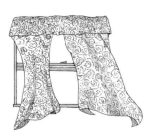 # Resources

Many excellent national organizations and resources are available to the family caregiver. These groups provide a broad spectrum of services, education, and information on subjects including elder care facilities, medical conditions, health care referral services, and caregiver support.

Locally, many valuable services are available for caregivers and their relatives, some of which are available at little or no cost. You may be eligible for having meals delivered to your home. Meals on Wheels is one example of such a service. You may be able to take advantage of transportation services that provide rides for seniors to stores, appointments, and social events. Churches and community agencies in your area may have volunteer companions who make regular visits or calls to help ease isolation and loneliness. Some churches or social service agencies offer help with household tasks and maintenance for people who live alone and cannot manage the tasks themselves. Adult day care centers offer a range of services including meals, social activity, and therapy. Some provide transportation to and from the center as well. Start your search for support and services locally, through your Area Agency on Aging, senior services, senior center, churches, and other community service agencies.

Caregiver Support

CaregiverZone
2855 Telegraph Avenue, Suite 601
Berkeley, CA 94705
(510) 981-5000
www.caregiverzone.com
Comprehensive Internet resource, including an online magazine, caregiver coping tools, virtual tours of eldercare facilities, medical and household products for older people.

Family Caregiver Alliance
690 Market Street, Suite 600
San Francisco, CA 94104.
(415) 434-3388
email: info@caregiver.org
http://www.caregiver.org
Web site with online caregiver support group, newsletter, and other resources.

Well Spouse Foundation
30 East 40th Street, Suite PH
New York, NY 10016
(800) 838-0879
(212) 685-8815
http://www.wellspouse.org
email: wellspouse@aol.com
Newsletter, support groups, email pen pals, regional activities.

National Family Caregivers Association
10605 Concord Street, Suite 501
Kensington, MD 20895-2504
(800) 896-3650
(301) 942-6430
info@nfcacares.org
http://www.nfcacares.org
Website contains list of recommended reading, information on national projects supporting family caregivers. Dues are $20 per year. Newsletter.

Eldercare Locator
(800) 677-1116
Locates local resources providing services to the elderly and protective services for domestic violence.

CAPS (Children of Aging Parents)
1609 Woodbourne Road, Suite 302-A
Levittown, PA 19057
(215) 945-6900 or (800)227-7294
http://www.careguide.net/

Children of Aging Parents (CAPS) is a nonprofit organization that provides information and emotional support to caregivers of older people. CAPS serves as a national clearinghouse for information on resources and issues dealing with older people.

Caregiver Survival Resources
http://www.caregiver911.com
A comprehensive listing of sources for general caregiving information and services for specific chronic illnesses.

Tad Publishing & Consulting Co.
www.caregiving.com
Caregiving support and newsletter

Communication

American Speech-Language-Hearing Association (ASHA)
10801 Rockville Pike
Rockville, MD 20852
(800) 638-8255 or (301) 897-8682
http://www.asha.org
http://www.audiology.org
Contact ASHA for a list of audiologists in your state. The website offer extensive information on hearing aids and assistive listening devices.

Self Help for Hard of Hearing People (SHHH)
7910 Woodmont Avenue, Suite 1200
Bethesda, MD 20814
(301) 657-2248

(301) 657-2249 (TTY)
Offers information about hearing loss and hearing aids.

AT&T Special Needs Center
(800) 872-3883 (TTY)

Nutrition

American Dietetic Association
(800) 366-1655, 10:00am-5:00pm ET weekdays
The ADA can help you locate a registered dietician in your
area.

Area Agency on Aging or
Cooperative Extension Service
Your local office may offer free counseling by a registered
dietician.

Incontinence

A+ Medical Products, Inc.
http://www.aplusmedical.com, 888-843-3334
Offers a female urinal.

American Urological Association
http://www.drylife.org
Urinary continence education, primarily for women.

Briggs Catalog
http://www.briggscorp.com, 800-247-2343
Bladder retraining assessment form, comfort pan, disposable and reusable incontinence products, urine drainage bag.

Buck & Buck Designs Catalog
http://www.buckandbuck.com
800-458-0600
Easy wear and care clothing for older people.

National Association for Continence (NAFC)
P.O. Box 8310
Spartanburg, SC 29305-8310
(864) 579-7900
(800) 252-3337
http://www.nafc.org
NAFC provides education, support, and management options for incontinence.

Fall Prevention

Area Agency on Aging

National Resource Center on Aging and Injury
College of Health and Human Services
San Diego State University
5500 Campanile Dr.
San Diego, CA 92182
(619) 594-6765
http://www.olderadultinjury.com
Website provides information on books, videos, articles, pamphlets, and websites related to prevention of injury in older adults.

American Association of Retired Persons (AARP)
601 E Street NW

Washington, DC 20049
1-800-424-3410
http://www.aarp.org
Ask for the booklet "The Do-Able Renewable Home"

National Association of Home Builders Research
Center
400 Prince George's Blvd
Upper Marlboro, MD 20774
(301) 249-4000
http://nahbrc.org
Produces publications including *Home Planning for Your Later Years and Retrofitting Houses for a Lifetime.*

Center for Universal Design
North Carolina State University
School of Design
Box 8613
Raleigh, NC 27695-8613
(919)515-3082 or 800-647-6777
E-mail: cud@ncsu.edu
http://www.design.ncsu.edu/cud
Founded by the National Institute on Disability and Reha-
bilitation Research (NIDRR), the CUD offers services in-
cluding information, referral service, technical design as-
sistance, and publications.

Elder Neglect and Abuse

National Center on Elder Abuse
810 1st St. NE, Suite 500

Washington, DC 20002
(202)682-2470
http://www.gwjapan.com/NCEA/
Fact sheets, laws, conferences, and phone numbers for reporting elder abuse are included, as well as links to other related sites.

Medical and Health Information

The Health Resource, Inc.
524 Locust Street
Conway, AR 72032
(501) 329-5272
Fax (501) 329-9489
(800) 949-0090
The Health Resource prepares individualized, comprehensive reports on specific medical conditions. The reports include descriptions of conventional and alternative treatments and information on current research, nutrition, self-help measures, specialists, and resource organizations. Reports on any non-cancer condition cost $275 and are 50-100 pages long; reports on any cancer condition are $375 and are 150-250 pages long.

Medcetera, Inc.
4515 Merrie Lane
Bellaire, TX 77401
(800) 748-6866 or (713) 664-3222
Fax (713) 666-6891

http://users.netropolis.net/pgeyer/default.htm
Customized research reports with current information on any medical condition from Medline, the world's largest medical database. Searches cost from $89-$135 and up.

Doctor's Guide to the Internet - Patient Edition
http: //www.pslgroup.com/PTGUIDE.HTM
Information for specific diseases and links to other Internet sites.

BOOKS

The Caregiver Helpbook: Powerful Tools for Caregiving, Vicki L. Schmall, Ph.D., Marilyn Cleland, R.N., Marilynn Sturdevant, R.N., M.S.W., L.C/S.W., 2000, Legacy Caregiver Services, 1015 NW 22nd Ave., N300, Portland, OR 97210 www.legacyhealth.org

When Aging Parents Can't Live Alone, Ellen F. Rubenson, M.S.W. 2000, Lowell House, 4255 West Touhy Ave., Lincolnwood, IL 60646-1975

Caregiving: The Spiritual Journey of Love, Loss, and Renewal, Beth Witrogen McLeod, 1999, John Wiley & Sons

Helping Yourself Help Others, Rosalynn Carter, Susan K. Golant, 1996, Time Books

Another Country: Navigating the Emotional Terrain of our Elders, Mary Bray Pipher, 1999, Riverhead Books

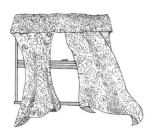

Glossary

Active Listening A communication skill used to show interest and involvement in what is being expressed. The listener pays close attention to the speaker and applies techniques such as paraphrasing, body language, and asking for explanation or more information.

Adverse Reaction Any new, unwanted, harmful, or unexpected response to a medication.

Airborne Contact Germs/microrganisms that are acquired by breathing dust particles or air droplets suspended in the air from someone sneezing, coughing, or talking.

Alzheimer's Disease An incurable, chronic degenerative disease characterized by memory loss and progressive mental and physical decline.

Aseptic Technique Methods used to prevent the spread of germs. Proper handwashing is an example of an aseptic technique.

Assistive Listening Devices Telephone amplifiers, infra-red headsets to amplify television programs, loud doorbell ringers, and other devices.

Audiologist A professional trained to evaluate hearing, identify impaired hearing, and determine the need for re-habilitation. The audiologist selects and fits a hearing aid if necessary.

Auto Touch Lamps Lamps that turn on when you touch any part of the lamp. They are helpful for people with arthritis or painful joints.

Axillary Temperature Taking the temperature under the armpit, or axilla.

Bed Protector A moisture-absorbent pad placed between the person and the bed to keep both skin and linens dry.

Blanching Normally, skin will turn white after it has been gently pressed. This is called blanching. On an area that is beginning to form a pressure ulcer, the reddened area of the skin does not blanch.

Blood Pressure Blood pressure measures the force that blood exerts against the walls of the blood vessels. Factors that can influence blood pressure readings include medications, exercise, emotions, pain, and stress.

Body Language Mannerisms, gestures, and postures that function as nonverbal communication.

Body Mechanics A set of rules that help maintain correct body posture during any movement. Good posture maintains the natural curves of the spine, helping to conserve energy and prevent muscle strain.

Brachial Artery The artery that runs on the inside of the elbow. It is commonly used for taking a blood pressure reading.

Brand Name The manufacturer's name of a drug. For instance, "Bayer" is a brand name for aspirin. Aspirin is the generic name.

Calorie The unit of measurement for the fuel or energy value of food. The amount of heat necessary to raise the temperature of 1 kilogram of water 1 degree C.

Case Manager The human services professional who oversees and plans every aspect of the patient's care. The case manager has extensive knowledge of the cost, quality, and availability of services in the community and makes arrangements for care based on a comprehensive assessment of the person's needs and resources.

Catheter A rubber tube used to drain and remove urine from the bladder.

Chronic Illness A continuous or recurring disease.

Closed Drainage System Consists of a catheter, connective tubing, and urine collection bag.

CPR: Cardiopulmonary Resuscitation A method used to restore breathing after the heart has stopped by applying rhythmic pressure on the chest and using mouth-to-mouth breathing assistance at regular intervals.

Dehydration Excessive loss of or lack of normal body fluid.

Dementia Progressive mental deterioration caused by brain damage or organic brain disease and characterized by irrational thoughts, communications, and behavior.

Depth Perception Three dimensional perception. The ability to recognize that an object is deep, as well as high and wide.

Diastolic Pressure The pressure felt in the artery when the heart is in a relaxed stage, filling with blood; the lower of the two numbers that measure blood pressure.

Direct Contact Germs spread by touching another person or handling body fluids.

Discharge Planner A hospital staff member who makes arrangements for the care of a patient upon release from the hospital, usually a professional nurse or social worker.

Disinfectant Cleaning solutions such as Lysol, Pinesol, or a 1:10 bleach/water solution that destroys germs/microrganisms.

Diuretic A drug or other substance that causes the body to eliminate fluids by frequent urination.

Draw Sheet A sheet placed in the middle third of the bed so that the person's torso and buttocks lie on it. It is used to help move the person with minimum friction to the skin.

Drugs Any substance that when taken into the living body may change one or more of its functions. Prescribed medications, over-the-counter medications, herbal preparations, natural remedies, alcohol, caffeine, and nicotine are all drugs.

Drug Interaction When one medicine reacts with another medicine.

Edema Swelling caused by excessive accumulation of water or fluid in body tissues.

Elder Abuse Harm caused to older people either physically, psychologically, or financially.

Enema A technique of introducing fluid into the rectum with the purpose of removing feces and gas from the rectum and colon.

Foley Catheter Also called an indwelling catheter, this kind of catheter is placed in the bladder to drain urine. It has a balloon at its tip that is inflated to keep it in place after insertion.

Foot Drop A condition that results in the inability to keep the foot in a normal flexed position.

Foot Board A device that is placed on the bed to keep a bed bound person's feet in an upright position. Used to prevent foot drop.

Foot Splint A form made for the foot to keep the foot in the proper flexed position. Used to prevent foot drop.

Friction A rubbing of the skin against a surface. Carelessly lifting or moving someone can cause friction.

Gait Belt A sturdy cloth strap, measuring about three inches wide and three feet long, placed around the waist to provide support when helping someone to walk or transfer from a wheelchair. Sometimes called a transfer belt.

Generic Name The standard accepted name for a drug, not protected by a trademark registration. Aspirin is an example of a generic name.

Germs Microorganisms capable of causing disease and infection.

Handwashing Technique The proper washing of hands. Handwashing is the most effective measure to prevent the spread of germs.

Hearing Aids Electronic amplifiers available in different types, from conventional to digital. Although hearing aids may improve hearing by amplifying sounds, they do not correct or restore damaged nerves in the ears.

Heimlich Maneuver A procedure for dislodging and expelling an object that is causing someone to choke.

Immune System The body's defense system. A weakened immune system cannot fight infections or disease as effectively as a strong immune system.

Incontinence The inability to control urination or defecation. Involuntary discharge of urine or feces.

Indirect Contact Germs that are spread by touching objects that have been touched by someone who is ill. Touching used dishes, soiled bed linens, soiled clothing, or used/soiled equipment are examples of indirect contact.

Intravenous (IV) The delivery of fluids, medications, or nutrients through a catheter inserted into a vein.

Medicare A federal health and hospitalization insurance program for people 65 or older, and for certain disabled people under the age of 65. Participation in Medicare is voluntary.

Microorganism A living plant or animal not visible to the naked eye.

Nonverbal Communication Communication without words through gestures, facial expressions, and other types of body language.

Output All of the fluids lost from the body that can be measured.

Over-the-Counter Drugs Medications you can buy without a doctor's prescription.

Passive Range of Motion Exercises Range of motion (ROM) exercises are designed to move muscles and joints through their complete natural range of motion. Passive range of motion exercises are done with the assistance of a caregiver because the person lacks sufficient strength to do the exercises independently.

Pathogen A harmful or disease-causing microorganism.

Perineal Area The area between the exterior genital organs and the anus.

Personal Protective Equipment (PPE) Equipment worn when providing care that prevents germs from entering the body, also known as protective barriers. Gloves, gowns and aprons, masks, and protective eye shields are protective equipment.

Physical Therapist A licensed professional who can teach correct body mechanics and improve the function of moving or walking for those affected by illness, injury, surgery, or disease.

Positioning Placing or moving a person into a position that allows and encourages functional activity and correct posture. Proper positioning should reduce the dangers of pressure sores, impaired breathing, and the stiffening, shrinking, and atrophy of muscles and tendons.

Pressure Points The areas of the body that receive the greatest amount of pressure when a person is lying in bed or in a wheelchair.

Pressure Ulcers A breakdown of the skin that becomes a chronic wound. Referred to as bedsores, dermal ulcers, and decubitus ulcers and caused by prolonged pressure on one spot.

Principles of Body Mechanics A set of rules that help maintain the natural curves of the back during any movement.

Prone A position in which the person is lying on the chest, stomach, and abdomen with the head turned to one side.

Pulse Throbbing felt in the arteries with each beat of the heart; the measurement of the number of heartbeats per minute.

Radial Artery The artery inside the wrist on the thumb

side; the most common place for checking a pulse.

Range of Motion Exercises (see passive range of motion exercises)

Reacher A mechanical device with a grip and trigger at one end and pincers at the other that can be used to extend the range of a person's reach.

Respite Care The word respite means relief, vacation, breather, pause, or time off. Respite care can be in-home or outside the home. An informal caregiver such as a church volunteer, friend or relative, may come to the home to relieve the primary caregiver. A professional caregiver may provide relief at an adult day care or respite center.

Sensorineural Hearing Loss A common type of hearing loss among the aging, caused by damage in the inner ear or nerve pathways to the brain. Causes may include past physical trauma, a history of hearing loss in the family, prior illnesses, medications, or noise.

Shear A condition that occurs when the pressure of movement pulls the skin in the opposite direction from the movement.

Side Effect A common, known response to a medication. Antihistamines, for example, are known to cause drowsiness.

Speech Reading Receiving cues about what is being said through lip movements, facial expression, body postures, and gestures.

Sphygmomanometer The traditional equipment used to

take blood pressure readings. Used with a stethoscope. The aneroid type uses a dial gauge and the mercury type uses a vertical gauge.

Sputum Material from the lungs coughed up and expelled through the mouth.

Sterile The absence of any germs/microrganisms.

Sublingual Medications Below or under the tongue. Medicine that is meant to be absorbed through the lining of the mouth.

Suppository A small plug of medication designed to be inserted into the rectum or vagina.

Sundowner's Syndrome The experience of some elderly people of severe confusion, anxiety, agitation, irritability, and even violent tendencies that come during a certain period at the end of the day, usually when the sun goes down.

Supine Lying on the back.

Systolic Pressure The pressure felt in the artery when the heart contracts and pumps the blood, the higher of the two numbers that measure blood pressure.

Tinnitis Ringing in the ears. Some people experience the sound of tinnitis as a whistle, while others may hear a sound like a foghorn. Tinnitis can be caused by medication as well as by too much caffeine or nicotine.

Tip Bars A feature located at the back of the wheelchair. Tip bars are used to tip the wheelchair up and down curbs.

Traction Relieving pressure on joints, muscles, or bones by pulling extremities into a new position, often with a traction device.

Transfer Moving someone from one surface area to another, for example, from the bed to the wheelchair.

Transfer Belt (see also Gait Belt) A sturdy cloth strap, measuring about three inches wide and three feet long, placed around the waist to assist a caregiver with lifting someone from and lowering someone into a sitting position. It can also be used for added support when helping someone who has difficulty walking.

Vector Spread Disease and germs that are spread from animals or insects. Encephalitis is an example of a disease that is spread from the mosquito.

Vehicle Spread Germs that are introduced into the body through contaminated drugs, food, water or blood products.

Vital Signs The important measured indicators of how the body is functioning: pulse, temperature, respiration, blood pressure, and intake and output of fluids.

Wheel Lock A feature on the wheel of the wheelchair that sets the wheelchair in a locked position. The wheelchair does not move when the lock is set.

Index

About Medifecta Healthcare Training

In 1995 Marion Karpinski, RN founded Healing Arts Communications (now Medifecta Healthcare Training) in response to witnessing families struggle to perform hospital-level duties at home with little or no training. Marion recognized that there was a pressing need for family caregiver education resources and teamed up with her husband, professional videographer Mike Karpinski to produce their first instructional video, Caring for Someone on Bedrest.

Since then, the team at Medifecta Healthcare Training has produced standardized training programs for family and professional caregivers and a series of DVDs on caregiving and communication topics.

The American Society on Aging honored the company in 2005 for "its work in providing exemplary programs and services that meet the needs of the aging population."

The National Alliance for Caregiving gave a 4-star rating to National Caregiver Training Program, an educational course for family caregivers. National Alliance for Caregiving has also given 4-star ratings to many of our DVD programs. Other groups who recognized the excellence of our materials include National Hospice Foundation, Video Librarian and National Mature Media.

We have developed excellent resources on Alzheimer's, aphasia, cultural competence, nutrition for older adults and many other important caregiver topics.

Our DVDs are available in an online viewing format, too, making it easy to learn at home or work.

Thousands of organizations rely upon our training materials to educate family and professional caregivers.

Please visit our website, www.medifecta.com, for information on all of our training materials or call us at 888-846-7008 for further information.